FOR REFERENCE

NOT TO BE TAKEN FROM THE ROOM

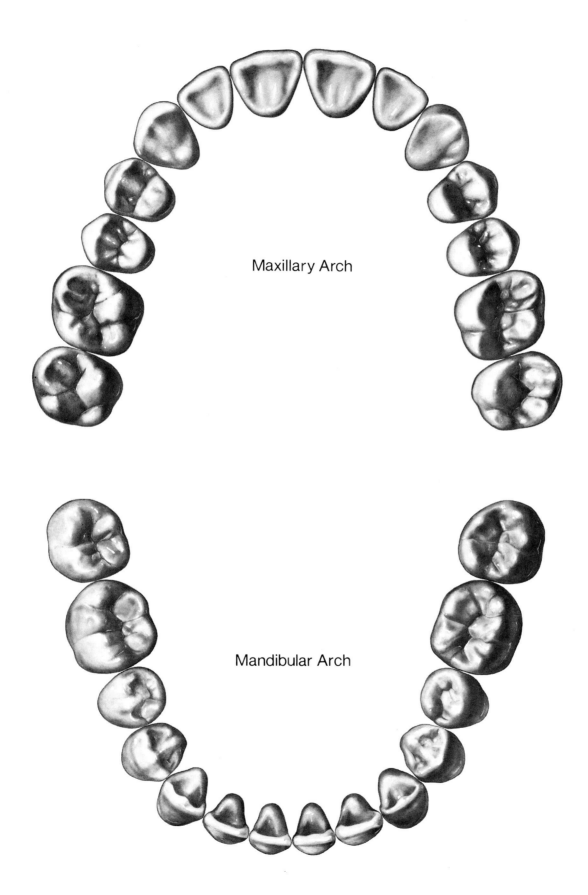

Maxillary Arch

Mandibular Arch

Major M. Ash, JR., B.S., D.D.S., M.S.

Professor and Chairman, Department of Occlusion and TMJ Clinic,
School of Dentistry, University of Michigan

FIFTH EDITION

W.B. SAUNDERS COMPANY

Philadelphia □ London □ Toronto □ Mexico City □ Rio de Janeiro □ Sydney □ Tokyo

Wheeler's **ATLAS OF**
TOOTH FORM

W. B. SAUNDERS COMPANY
Harcourt Brace Jovanovich, Inc.

The Curtis Center
Independence Square West
Philadelphia, PA 19106

Library of Congress Cataloging in Publication Data
Wheeler, Russell C. (Russell Charles)
Wheeler's An atlas of tooth form.
Rev. ed. of: Atlas of tooth form. 4th ed. 1969.
1. Teeth. 2. Dentures. I. Ash, Major M. II. Wheeler, Russell C. (Russell Charles). Atlas of tooth form. 4th ed. III. Title. IV. Title: Atlas of tooth form. [DNLM: 1. Tooth—Anatomy and histology—Atlases. 2. Dental prosthesis—Laboratory manuals. WU 17 W564a]
RK656.W45 1984   611'.314   83-20383
ISBN 0-7216-1277-6

Wheeler's An Atlas of Tooth Form   ISBN   0-7216-1277-6

Last digit is the print number: 9   8   7   6   5

Preface to the Fifth Edition

This edition of *An Atlas of Tooth Form* is dedicated to Dr. Russell C. Wheeler, who introduced so many of us to the "art" and science of dental anatomy. His contributions to an understanding of the form and function of the teeth are too numerous to be listed, but this atlas and the textbook *Dental Anatomy, Physiology and Occlusion* reflect a dedication to the subject seldom equaled in any field of endeavor.

The organization of the *Atlas* is evident from its table of contents, which represents an outline of the material considered. Those minor changes or additions that have been made reflect an attempt to make this book consistent with recent developments in concepts of form and function. These concepts are discussed in more detail in the new sixth edition of *Dental Anatomy, Physiology and Occlusion.*

A number of new illustrations have been introduced, especially where ideas concerning dental illustration have changed since the last edition.

This book is written primarily for the student and intended to give him or her a concept of dental anatomy useful in dentistry or subjects ancillary to dentistry. It attempts to bridge the gap between basic and applied knowledge and to provide those experiences in learning that are essential for an appreciation of form and function in dental anatomy and for the restoration of lost tooth structures.

MAJOR M. ASH

Contents

Chapter 1

Nomenclature and General Considerations........................... 1
  Surfaces and Ridges 4
  Other Landmarks 5
  Division into Thirds 8

Chapter 2

Dental Physiology and Tooth Form..................................... 8
  Proximal Contact Areas 12
  Interproximal Spaces 13
  Occlusal (Incisal) Thirds... 14
  Embrasures and Escapement 15
  Facial and Lingual Contours (Protective)........................... 17
  Curvatures of the Cervical Line on Mesial and
      Distal Surfaces 18

Chapter 3

Drawing to Scale and Carving Models to Scale......................... 19

Chapter 4

Plan for the Laboratory Course 24

Chapter 5

Drawing... 25
  Measurements of the Teeth 26
  Use of Measurement Table in Outlining Drawings
      and Carvings 27
  Methods of Calibrating an Anterior Tooth 28
  Method of Calibrating a Posterior Tooth 29

Chapter 6

Individual Tooth Form, Maxillary Arch................................ 32
  Maxillary Central Incisor 32

Maxillary Lateral Incisor.. 35
Maxillary Canine.. 36
Maxillary First Premolar.. 41
Maxillary Second Premolar.. 45
Maxillary First Molar... 47
Maxillary Second Molar... 52
Maxillary Third Molar... 55

Chapter 7

Individual Tooth Form, Mandibular Arch 57
Mandibular Central Incisor.. 57
Mandibular Lateral Incisor 61
Mandibular Canine 61
Mandibular First Premolar 63
Mandibular Second Premolar 67
Mandibular First Molar 69
Mandibular Second Molar 72
Mandibular Third Molar 74

Chapter 8

Plaster Sculpture.. 76
Laboratory Technique Described and Illustrated 76
Maxillary Right Central Incisor 85
Maxillary Right Lateral Incisor 86
Maxillary Right Canine ......,... 87
Maxillary Right First Premolar 88
Maxillary Right Second Premolar.. 89
Maxillary Right First Molar 90
Maxillary Right Second Molar 91
Mandibular Right Central Incisor 92
Mandibular Right Lateral Incisor... 93
Mandibular Right Canine.. 94
Mandibular Right First Premolar.. 95
Mandibular Right Second Premolar.. 96
Mandibular Right First Molar 98
Mandibular Right Second Molar... 99

Chapter 9

Carving Teeth Normal Size 100
Carving in Wax 100
Carving in Ivorine 101

Chapter 10

Illustrations to Be Used for Reference Purposes in Carving............ 109

Chapter 11

Arrangement of the Teeth and Occlusion................................. 126
Functional Form of the Teeth at Their Incisal and
    Occlusal Thirds 127

Dental Arch Formation (Alignment) 131
Compensating Curvature of the Dental Arches 132
Contact Relations of the Teeth.................................... 133
Occlusal Contact and Intercusp Relations........................... 135

Chapter 12

The Deciduous Teeth 138
Description of the Deciduous Teeth............................... 140
    Incisors and Canines... 140
    Molars 145
The Occlusion of the Deciduous Teeth............................. 155
Details of Occlusion 157

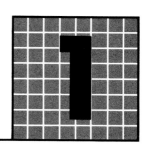

Nomenclature and General Considerations

In order to obtain a comprehensive view of any subject, one must know the nomenclature and have a general understanding of what the subject includes. All dentists and everyone interested in the practice of dentistry must speak a common language.

"An Atlas of Tooth Form" has to do with the macroscopic or gross anatomy of the human teeth, their contact with each other in the dental arches, their alignment and their occlusion. Already, two terms have been used which need explanation: *alignment* is used to denote the way the teeth are arranged in the dental arches—*maxillary* and *mandibular*; *occlusion* is the term used to denote the contact of the teeth of the two arches when the jaws are closed. The *maxilla* is the upper jaw; the *mandible,* the lower jaw; hence, *maxillary* and *mandibular*.

Chapters 1 through 11 of this book are concerned with the permanent or secondary teeth. In Figure 1, the permanent teeth are named.

Each tooth has a *crown* and *root* portion. The surface of the crown is made up of *enamel,* and the surface of the root is made up of *cementum*. The crown and root join at the *cementoenamel junction*. This junction, also called the cervical line (Fig. 2), is plainly visible on a specimen tooth. The main bulk of the tooth, under enamel and cementum, is composed of *dentin,* which is seen in a cross section (Fig. 3).

The *crown* of an incisor tooth has an incisal *ridge* or edge; the crown of a canine has a single *cusp*; the crowns of premolars and molars have two or more cusps. Incisal ridges and cusps form the cutting surfaces on tooth crowns.

The *root* of the tooth may be *single,* with one apex or terminal end as found in normal *anterior* teeth and some of the premolars; or *multiple,* with a *bifurcation* or *trifurcation* dividing the root into two or more parts with their apices or terminal ends, as found ordinarily on all molars and on some premolars.

The *root* of the tooth is attached by connective tissue fibers to the bony process of the jaw, holding the tooth firmly in its position relative to the others in the *dental arch*. The portion of the jaw that serves as a support for the tooth is called the *alveolar process*. The tooth "socket" in which the tooth rests is called the *alveolus* (plural, *alveoli*).

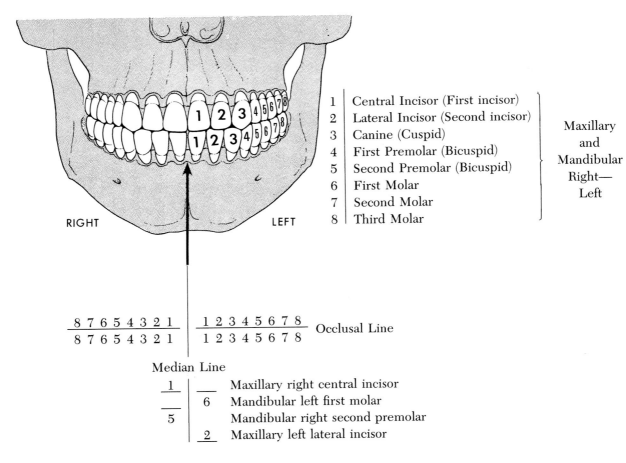

1	Central Incisor (First incisor)
2	Lateral Incisor (Second incisor)
3	Canine (Cuspid)
4	First Premolar (Bicuspid)
5	Second Premolar (Bicuspid)
6	First Molar
7	Second Molar
8	Third Molar

Maxillary and Mandibular Right— Left

RIGHT   LEFT

$$\frac{8\ 7\ 6\ 5\ 4\ 3\ 2\ 1}{8\ 7\ 6\ 5\ 4\ 3\ 2\ 1} \Big| \frac{1\ 2\ 3\ 4\ 5\ 6\ 7\ 8}{1\ 2\ 3\ 4\ 5\ 6\ 7\ 8} \text{ Occlusal Line}$$

Median Line

$\underline{1}$		Maxillary right central incisor
	6	Mandibular left first molar
$\overline{5}$		Mandibular right second premolar
	$\underline{2}$	Maxillary left lateral incisor

DIAGNOSIS CHART CODE
(Palmer Notation)*

The Palmer Notation is the simplest and the most universally used code for dental records. Only eight different names of teeth need be remembered. A number within a directionally oriented right angle will identify the tooth and establish its location as maxillary, mandibular, right or left. Example:—6, Maxillary Left first molar.

PATIENT FACES OPERATOR

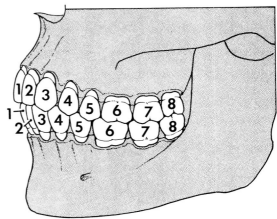

Figure 1. Naming the teeth, with an illustration of the method of using the Palmer Notation or code for dental records.

---

*"Palmer's Dental Notation," Dental Cosmos, Vol. 33, Pages 194–198, 1891.

The crown is never covered by bone tissue after it is fully erupted, but in children it is partly covered at the *cervical third* by soft tissue of the mouth known as the *gingiva* or *gingival tissue*, or *gum tissue*.

All of the foundation tissues surrounding the teeth make up the *periodontium*.

Figure 2. Maxillary central incisor (labial aspect). *A*, Apex of root; *R*, root; *CL*, cervical line; *C*, crown; *IE*, incisal edge.

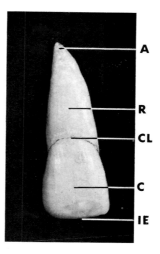

Figure 3. Schematic drawings of cross sections of an anterior and a posterior tooth. *A*, Anterior tooth. *A*, Apex; *AF*, apical foramen; *SC*, supplementary canal; *C*, cementum; *PM*, periodontal membrane; *B*, bone; *PC*, pulp canal; *G*, gingiva; *GC*, gingival sulcus; *GM*, gingival margin; *PCH*, pulp chamber; *D*, dentin; *E*, enamel; *CR*, crown; *R*, root. *B*, Posterior tooth. *A*, Apices; *PC*, pulp canal; *PCH*, pulp chamber; *PH*, pulp horn; *F*, fissure; *CU*, cusp; *CEJ*, cementoenamel junction; *BI*, bifurcation of roots.

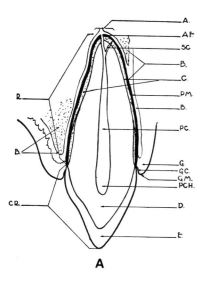

A

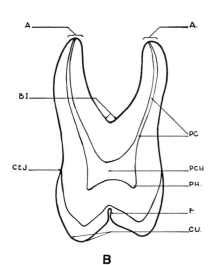

B

SURFACES AND RIDGES

The crowns of the incisors and canines have four surfaces and a ridge, and the crowns of the premolars and molars have five surfaces. The surfaces are named according to their positions and uses (Fig. 4). Central and lateral incisors and canines are called *anterior teeth*; premolars and molars are called *posterior teeth*. Those surfaces of the incisors and canines facing toward the lips are called *labial surfaces*; those surfaces of the premolars and molars facing toward the cheek are called *buccal surfaces*. When labial and buccal surfaces are spoken of collectively, they are called *facial surfaces*. All surfaces facing toward the tongue are called *lingual surfaces*. The surfaces of the teeth which come in contact with those in the opposite jaw during the act of closure (called *occlusion*) are called *occlusal surfaces*. In order to be more specific, these surfaces on the incisors and canines are called *incisal surfaces*.

The surfaces of the teeth which face or lie adjacent to teeth in the same dental arch are called *proximal surfaces*. The proximal surfaces are more clearly defined by the terms *mesial* and *distal*. These terms have special reference to the position of the surface relative to the *median line* of the dental arch. This line passes between the central incisors at their point of contact with each other in both dental arches. Those proximal surfaces which, following the curve of the arch, are faced toward the median line, are called *mesial surfaces*, and those most distant from the median line are called *distal surfaces*.

Four teeth have mesial surfaces which contact each other: the maxillary and mandibular central incisors. In all other instances the mesial surface of one tooth contacts the distal surface of its neighbor. By the same token, a distal surface of one tooth contacts the mesial surface of another, except for

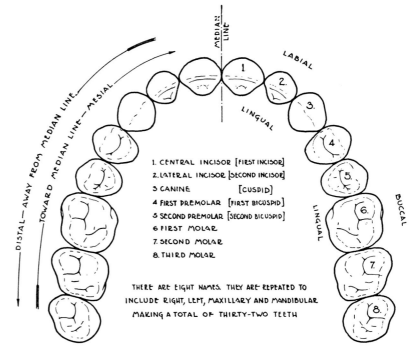

1. CENTRAL INCISOR [FIRST INCISOR]
2. LATERAL INCISOR [SECOND INCISOR]
3. CANINE   [CUSPID]
4. FIRST PREMOLAR [FIRST BICUSPID]
5. SECOND PREMOLAR [SECOND BICUSPID]
6. FIRST MOLAR
7. SECOND MOLAR
8. THIRD MOLAR

THERE ARE EIGHT NAMES. THEY ARE REPEATED TO INCLUDE RIGHT, LEFT, MAXILLARY AND MANDIBULAR MAKING A TOTAL OF THIRTY-TWO TEETH

Figure 4. Names and numbers of teeth and relationship to median line of the dental arches.

distal surfaces of the last teeth in both arches, usually second or third molars. The area of the mesial or distal surface of a tooth which comes in contact with its neighbor in the arch is called the *contact area*.

OTHER LANDMARKS

In order to study an individual tooth intelligently one must be able to recognize all landmarks of importance by name (Figs. 5, 6, 7, 8, 9, 10). Therefore, at this point, it will be necessary to become familiar with additional terms such as:

cusp	triangular ridge	sulcus
cingulum	transverse ridge	developmental groove
ridge	oblique ridge	supplemental groove
marginal ridge	fossa	pit

Figure 5. Maxillary right central incisor—lingual aspect—incial aspect. *CL,* Cervical line; *C,* cingulum; *MMR,* mesial marginal ridge; *LIE* (1) labioincisal edge; *LIE* (2), linguoincisal edge; *LF,* lingual fossa; *DMR,* distal marginal ridge.

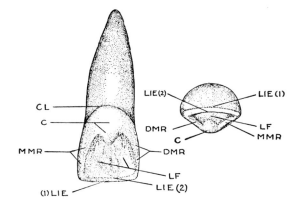

A *cusp* is an elevation on the crown of a tooth making up a divisional part of the occlusal surface (Fig. 3 *B*).

A *cingulum* is the lingual lobe of an anterior tooth. It makes up the bulk of the cervical third of the lingual surface. Its convexity mesiodistally resembles a girdle (Latin *cingulum*—girdle) encircling the lingual surface at the cervical third (Fig. 5).

A *ridge* is any linear elevation on the surface of a tooth and is named according to its location or form: *buccal* ridge, *incisal* ridge, *marginal* ridge, and so on.

Marginal ridges are those rounded borders of the enamel which form the margins of the occlusal surfaces of premolars and molars, mesially and distally, and the mesial and distal margins of the incisors and canines lingually.

Triangular ridges are those ridges which descend from the tips of the cusps of molars and premolars toward the central part of the occlusal surfaces. They are so named because the slopes of each side of the ridge are inclined to resemble two sides of a triangle. They are named after the cusps to which they belong: *triangular ridge of the buccal cusp of the maxillary first premolar*, and so on (Fig. 6).

When a buccal and a lingual triangular ridge join, they form a *transverse ridge*, the union of two triangular ridges crossing transversely the surface of a posterior tooth.

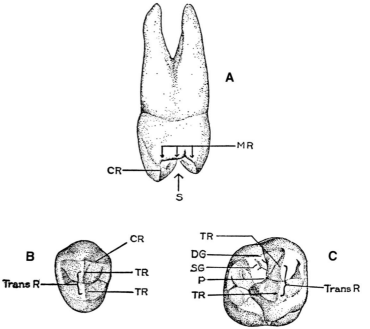

Figure 6. *A*, Mesial view of a maxillary first premolar. *S*, Sulcus traversing occlusal surface; *MR*, marginal ridge; *CR*, cusp ridge.

B, Occlusal view of maxillary first premolar. *CR*, Cusp ridge; *TR*, triangular ridges; *Trans R*, transverse ridge, formed by two triangular ridges crossing the tooth transversely.

C, Occlusal view of a maxillary first molar. *TR*, Triangular ridge; *DG*, developmental groove; *SG*, supplemental groove; *P*, pit, formed by junction of developmental grooves; *TR*, triangular ridge; *Trans R*, transverse ridge.

The *oblique ridge* is formed by the union of the triangular ridge of the distobuccal cusp and the distal cusp ridge of the mesiolingual cusp of maxillary molars, especially the maxillary first molar (see Fig. 8).

A *fossa* is an irregular, rounded depression or concavity found on the surface of a tooth. *Lingual* fossae are found upon the lingual surface of incisors. *Central* fossae are found upon the occlusal surface of molars and are formed by the converging of ridges terminating at a central point in the bottom of the depression where there is a junction of grooves. *Triangular* fossae are found on molars and premolars on the occlusal surfaces mesial or distal to marginal ridges, as the case may be (Fig. 7); they are sometimes found on the lingual surfaces of maxillary incisors at the edge of the lingual fossae where the marginal ridge and the cingulum meet (Fig. 5).

A *sulcus* is a long depression or valley in the surface of a tooth between ridges and cusps, the inclines of which meet at an angle. A sulcus has a developmental groove at the junction of its inclines. (The term *sulcus* must not be confused with the term *groove*. Compare Figure 6 with Figure 7.)

A *developmental groove* is a shallow groove or line on a tooth, probably denoting evidence of coalescence between the primary parts of the crown or root. A *supplemental groove* is also a shallow linear depression on the surface of a tooth, but it is usually less distinct and more variable than a developmental groove and does not mark the junction of primary parts. *Buccal* and *lingual grooves* are developmental grooves found on the buccal and lingual surfaces of posterior teeth.

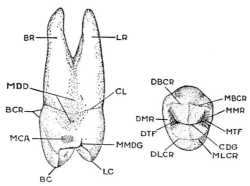

Figure 7. Maxillary right first premolar—mesial aspect—occlusal aspect. *LR*, Lingual root; *CL*, cervical line; *MMDG*, mesial marginal developmental groove; *LC*, lingual cusp; *BC*, buccal cusp; *MCA*, mesial contact area; *BCR*, buccal cervical ridge; *MDD*, mesial developmental depression; *BR*, buccal root; *MBCR*, mesiobuccal cusp ridge; *MMR*, mesial marginal ridge; *MTF*, mesial triangular fossa (shaded area); *CDG*, central developmental groove; *MLCR*, mesiolingual cusp ridge; *DLCR*, distolingual cusp ridge; *DTF*, distal triangular fossa; *DMR*, distal marginal ridge; *DBCR*, distobuccal cusp ridge.

Figure 8. Maxillary first molar—occlusal landmarks. *MBCR*, Mesiobuccal cusp ridge; *CF*, central fossa (shaded area); *MTF*, mesial triangular fossa (shaded area); *MMR*, mesial marginal ridge; *MLCR*, mesiolingual cusp ridge; *OR*, oblique ridge; *DLCR*, distolingual cusp ridge; *DF*, distal fossa; *DTF*, distal triangular fossa (shaded area); *DMR*, distal marginal ridge; *DBCR*, distobuccal cusp ridge.

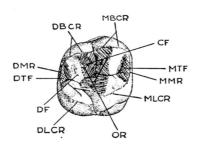

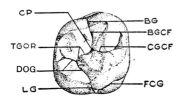

Figure 9. Maxillary first molar—occlusal aspect—developmental grooves. *BG*, Buccal groove; *BGCF*, buccal groove of central fossa; *CGCF*, central groove of central fossa; *FCG*, fifth cusp groove; *LG*, lingual groove; *DOG*, distal oblique groove; *TGOR*, transverse groove of oblique ridge; *CP*, central pit.

Figure 10. Maxillary first molar—distal aspect. *DBR*, Distobuccal root; *MBR*, mesiobuccal root; *BDG*, buccal developmental groove; *DBC*, distobuccal cusp; *DMR*, distal marginal ridge; *DLC*, distolingual cusp; *DCA*, distal contact area; *CL*, cervical line; *LR*, lingual root.

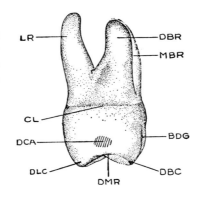

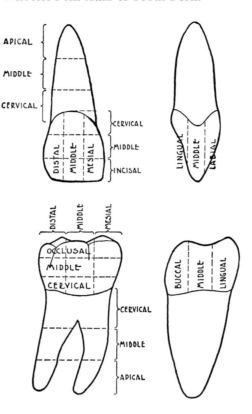

Figure 11. Division into thirds.

Pit is a term used to describe an important landmark found on the occlusal surfaces of molars where developmental grooves cross or join (i.e., the *central pit* of the mandibular first molar where developmental grooves join in the central fossa). The term "pit" is often associated with the term "fissure" in old terminology. They were used simultaneously to denote *normal landmarks* (meaning pits and grooves) and *faulty formation*, which should be called *pit-faults* and *fissures*. The term *fissure* means *linear fault*; it should not be used when the term "groove" (developmental) is intended.

DIVISION INTO THIRDS

For purposes of description and comparison, each surface of a tooth is divided into *thirds*. This makes it possible to visualize designated points specifically.

When the surfaces of the crown and root portions are divided into *thirds*, these thirds are named in accordance with the areas they approximate. Looking at the tooth from the *labial* or *buccal* aspect, one sees that the crown and root may be divided into thirds from the incisal or occlusal surface of the crown to the apex of the root (Fig. 11). The *crown* may be divided into an incisal or occlusal third, middle third and cervical third, etc.

The crown may be divided into thirds in three directions: inciso- or occlusocervically, mesiodistally, or labio- or buccolingually. Mesiodistally it is divided into the mesial, middle and distal thirds. Labio- or buccolingually it is divided into labial or buccal, middle and lingual thirds. Each of the five surfaces or aspects of a crown may be marked off in thirds in making a survey of any aspect. There will be one middle third and two other thirds which are named according to the area they approach, such as cervical, occlusal, mesial, or lingual.

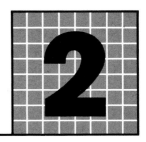

Dental Physiology and Tooth Form

Physiology is the study of the functions of organs and parts during life, as distinct from *anatomy*, which deals with their structure. The study of tooth form includes both subjects. The anatomic form of a tooth is also its functional form.

Teeth are unique among body tissues in that their static outside form (macroscopic) is functional. In addition, they are incapable of readaptation to new conditions and are incapable of having their structure rebuilt by the body when it has been injured or destroyed by wear or accident.

Human teeth perform two major functions during life: (1) they incise and reduce food material during mastication, and (2) they help to sustain themselves in the dental arches by assisting in the development and protection of the tissues that support them. Protection of the investing tissues and stabilization of the alignment are provided by the normal form of the individual teeth, by their proper alignment with others in the same jaw, by normal development of the jaws and by the proper relation of one jaw to the other during functional movements.

Generally speaking, the form of the tooth crowns may be drawn within two geometric concepts: (1) the facial or lingual aspects may be outlined within trapezoids of various dimensions (Fig. 13), and (2) the mesial and distal aspects of all tooth crowns may be outlined within triangles or multiples of overlapping triangles. These aspects show the tapered effect of tooth crowns, which design assists in the biting and penetration of the food (Fig. 14).

Figure 13 illustrates the following fundamentals of form:

1. Interproximal spaces accommodate interproximal gingival tissue.

2. Spacing between the roots of one tooth and those of others allows sufficient bone tissue for a foundation or investment for the teeth and a supporting structure required to hold up gingival tissue to a normal level. Sufficient circulation of blood to the parts would be impossible without this appropriate spacing.

3. Each tooth crown in the dental arches must be in contact at some point with its neighbor, or neighbors, to protect the interproximal gingival tissue from trauma during mastication. The contact of one tooth with another in the arch tends to insure their relative positions through mutual support.

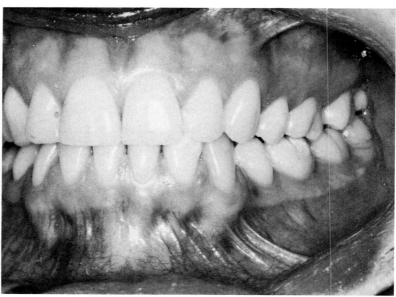

Figure 12. Relationship of teeth in centric occlusion, which is the terminal position of the chewing stroke and frequently in swallowing.

4. Each tooth in the dental arch has two antagonists in the opposing arch, excepting the mandibular central incisor and the maxillary third molar. In the event of loss of any tooth, this arrangement tends to prevent elongation of antagonists and helps to stabilize the remaining teeth over a longer period than would be likely if each tooth had a single antagonist.

Actually, of course, the form of tooth crowns is not so simple as the schematic drawings of fundamental form just described. Dental physiology is a subject quite extensive, and no attempt will be made to cover it here. *However, it is necessary that the student realize that the study of tooth form, drawing and carving, and tooth restoration is a scientific endeavor and not an art course.*

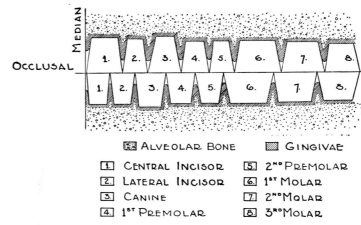

Figure 13. Schematic drawing of labial and buccal aspects of the teeth. This geometric concept illustrates the teeth as trapezoids of various dimensions. Note the relations of each tooth to its opposing tooth or teeth in the opposite arch. Each tooth has two antagonists except number 1 below and number 8 above.

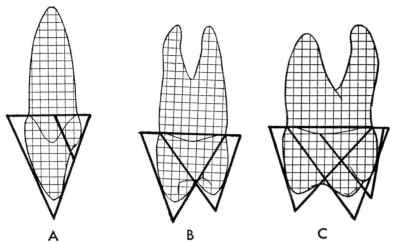

A   B   C

Figure 14. The functional form of the teeth when outlined schematically from the mesial or distal aspects is that of the fusion of two or three cones. *A,* Maxillary incisor; *B,* maxillary premolar; *C,* maxillary first molar. Note that the major portion of the incisor in view is made up of one cone or lobe.

A study of the form of tooth crowns must include the following:
1. Proximal contact areas
2. Interproximal spaces (formed by proximal surfaces in contact)
3. Occlusal (incisal) thirds
4. Embrasures and escapement
5. Facial and lingual contours (protective)
6. Curvatures of the cervical line on mesial and distal surfaces (cemento-enamel junction)

The above headings include the form, which has a direct or primary bearing on the protection of the *periodontium.* Many other details of tooth form have an indirect bearing on the stability of the teeth through their contribution to the maintenance of efficiency during function. Some of these details are cusp forms, the proportions of various measurements of the crowns and root, root form and anchorage, and angles at which teeth are set in the jaws.

Further observation of the details of tooth form soon establishes another important fact: from all aspects, when well-formed teeth are in normal alignment with normal gingival attachment (Fig. 15), they are remarkably

Figure 15. Normal, healthy gums, showing the interdental tissue papillae reaching well up into the embrasures. Subject is 65 years of age.

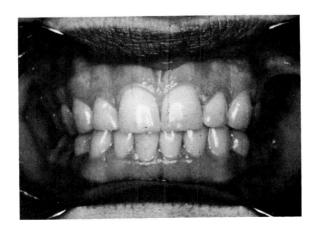

"self-cleansing." The smooth, rounded form of the teeth contributes toward proper dental hygiene when assisted by the brushing activity of tongue and cheeks and by the flushing action of saliva along with the intake of fluids, plus the friction of food material during the functional activity of mastication.

PROXIMAL CONTACT AREAS

Normally, there must be a positive contact relation mesially and distally of one tooth with another in each dental arch. Although the areas of contact are small, they are *areas* and not mere points of contact (Fig. 16). Only perfect spheres would approach a point contact when touching each other.

The contact areas are important functionally because they are protective. The proper contact relation between neighboring teeth does two things: (1) it serves to keep food from being trapped between the teeth, and (2) it helps to stabilize the dental arches by the combined anchorage of all the teeth in either arch in positive contact with each other.

Proper contact form will be learned through the study of various aspects of the teeth and by clinical evaluation (Fig. 17). Certain crests of curvature

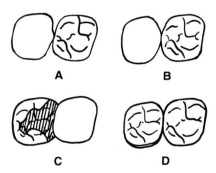

Figure 16. *A,* The projection of a point contact, as in a faulty restoration. This arrangement would not reproduce normal contact form or embrasure form. *B,* The contact is better than in *A,* but the supplementary embrasure form is faulty. *C,* Contact area is too great, with insuffucient embrasure opening, buccal and lingual. *D,* Normal contact and embrasure form.

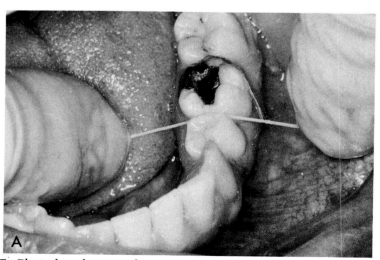

Figure 17. Clinical evaluation of contact area for "tightness" and smoothness using dental floss (*A*). "Tearing" of floss as shown may be related to a carious lesion (*B*).
Illustration continued on opposite page

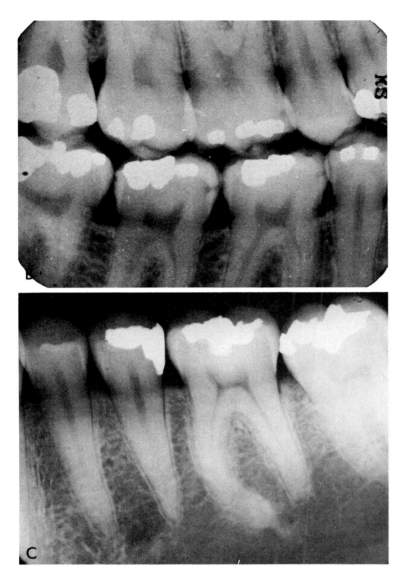

Figure 17 *Continued.* An "open" contact as shown in *C* would not impede the entry of floss. Such an open contact may lead to food impaction.

from facial, lingual and occlusal aspects will outline the contact areas. (See marginal illustrations on pages 34 to 73.)

INTERPROXIMAL SPACES

The interproximal spaces between the teeth are triangle-shaped spaces normally filled by *gingival tissue*. The base of the triangle is the alveolar process, the sides of the triangle are the proximal surfaces of the contacting teeth, and the apex of the triangle is in the area of contact. The form of the interproximal space will vary with the form of the teeth in contact and will depend also upon the relative position of the contact areas (Figs. 18 and 19).

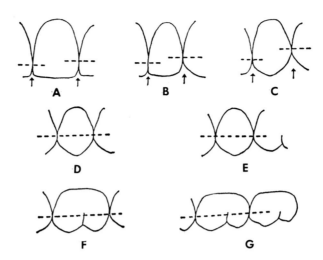

Figure 18. Outline drawings of the maxillary teeth in contact, with dotted lines bisecting the contact areas at the various levels as found normally. Arrows point to embrasure spaces. *A*, Central and lateral incisors; *B*, central and lateral incisors and canine; *C*, lateral incisor, canine and first premolar; *D*, canine, first and second premolars; *E*, first and second premolars and first molar; *F*, second premolar, first molar and second molar; *G*, first, second and third molars.

Figure 19. Contact levels found normally on mandibular teeth. Arrows point to embrasure spaces. *A*, Central and lateral incisors; *B*, central and lateral incisors and canine; *C*, lateral incisor, canine and first premolar; *D*, canine, first and second premolars; *E*, first and second premolars and first molar; *F*, second premolar, first and second molars; *G*, first, second and third molars.

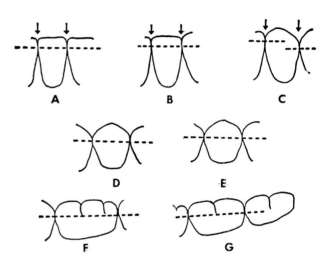

OCCLUSAL (INCISAL) THIRDS

When the teeth in the mandibular arch come into contact with the teeth of the maxillary arch in any functional relation during the various mandibular movements, *occlusion* is accomplished.

The occlusal thirds of the tooth crowns represent the "working" surfaces (Figs. 132, 133). These hard surfaces, when brought together with considerable jaw force, serve to reduce food material during mastication. This is the primary function of the teeth, of course, but remember that *the major portion of the tooth crown and root is designed for maintenance, directly or indirectly.*

The occlusal thirds also have an indirect bearing on maintenance. In addition to their ability to cut and crush food material, the teeth are stabilized by the efficiency of the occlusal thirds during this process. The efficiency of the curved occlusal surfaces as cutters with associated escapement spaces reduces forces brought to bear on the teeth, thereby insuring their positions in the arches.

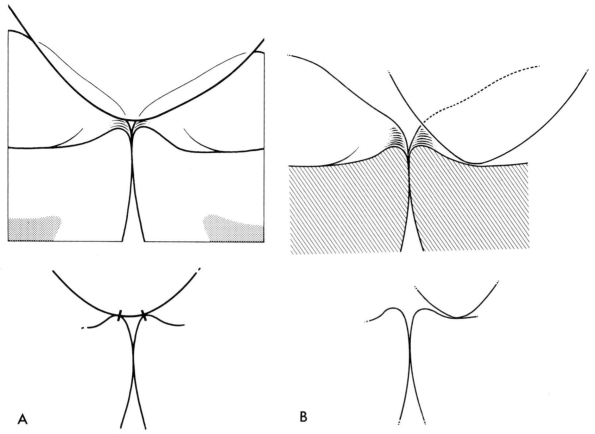

Figure 20. Possible relationship between cusp tip and marginal ridges forming embrasure space. *A*, Cusp tip occluding on approximating marginal ridges. *B*, Cusp tip occluding in distal fossa. Cusp tip may occlude on a single marginal ridge also in the natural dentition.

EMBRASURES AND ESCAPEMENT

Escapement spaces are provided in the teeth by the form of the cusps and ridges, the sulci and developmental grooves, and the interdental spaces called *embrasures* (Figs. 20 and 21). Most of the escapement, and consequent reduction of force against the teeth during mastication, is provided by the embrasures which open up all around the contact areas, occlusally, facially and lingually. The curved contacting surfaces of teeth opposing one another in occlusion allow escapement of food around the point of contact (Figs. 22, 23).

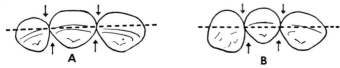

Figure 21. Outline drawings of the maxillary teeth from the incisal and occlusal aspects with broken lines bisecting the contact areas. These illustrations show the relative positions of the contact areas labiolingually and buccolingually. Arrows point to *embrasure* spaces. *A*, Central incisors and lateral incisor. *B*, Central and lateral incisor and canine.

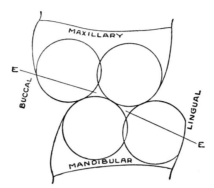

Figure 22. Schematic drawing of the mesial aspect of first molars in occlusion, illustrating the cusp forms as perfect circles. With this arrangement, escapement spaces would be larger, but the centric occlusal relation would be too unstable and the cusps would be too flat. *E*, Escapement spaces.

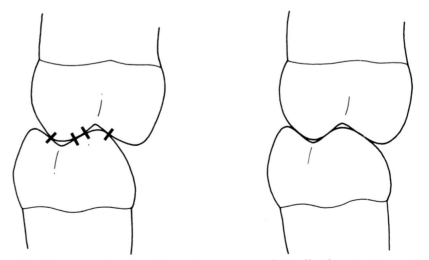

Figure 23. Schematic drawing illustrating more realistically than in Figure 22 the occlusal contact relations and escapement spaces.

FACIAL AND LINGUAL CONTOURS

It will be found that the tooth crowns, when viewed from mesial or distal aspects, have rather uniform curvatures at the cervical thirds and at the middle thirds labially or buccally and lingually, depending upon the teeth under consideration.

Since these contours are so constant, they must be recognized as having considerable physiologic importance. A major consideration is that the form should be conducive to the maintenance of good oral hygiene and free from trauma, for example, food impaction (Fig. 24).

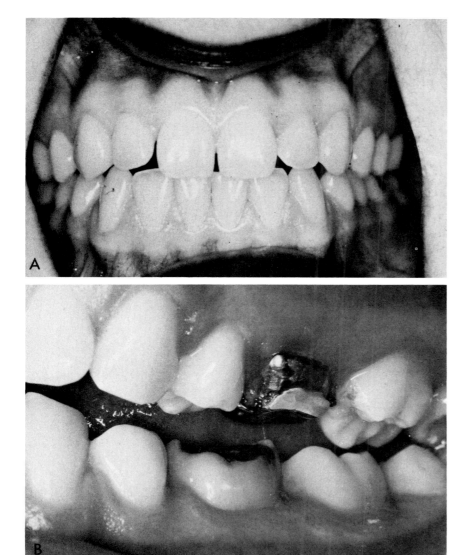

Figure 24. Gingival contours. *A,* Healthy gingivae in a patient with good oral hygiene. *B,* Gingivitis associated with temporary restoration with poor functional form, which contributes to retention of bacterial plaque and difficulty in maintaining oral hygiene.

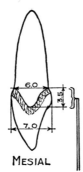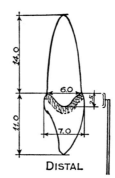

MESIAL   DISTAL

Figure 25. Curvatures of the cervical line (cementoenamel junction) mesially and distally on the maxillary central incisor, demonstrating the points of measurement in determining the relation between the curvature of the cervical line mesially and distally. Other points of measurement of the crown and root, when the student observes the mesial and distal aspects, are outlined. The shaded area in the form of a band on the enamel follows the cervical curvature and represents the epithelial attachment of gingival tissue to the enamel of the crown.

CURVATURES OF THE CERVICAL LINE
ON MESIAL AND DISTAL SURFACES
(Cementoenamel Junction)

The height of normal gingival tissue between the teeth (that is, mesial and distal on each tooth) is directly dependent upon the height of soft tissue attachment (epithelial). Normal attachment follows the curvature of the cemento-enamel junction. This statement does not mean that the epithelial attachment and the cervical line are at the same level (Fig. 25.)

Therefore, the curvature of the cementoenamel junction has physiologic as well as anatomic significance. Anatomically, the cementoenamel junction divides the crown and root and it will be referred to mostly as the *cervical line*.

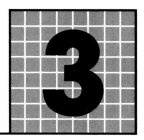

Drawing to Scale and Carving Models to Scale

Since form and function are allied so closely, it is necessary that the student be familiar with every detail in dental anatomy. If tooth restoration, either whole or in part, is to be done accurately, it is necessary to study the form of individual teeth and the relationship of the teeth to each other in the same arch and to the teeth in the opposing arch.

With greater accuracy in restoration in mind, an attempt was started some years ago to rationalize the teaching of tooth form by means of drawing to scale and carving to scale. When studying the form of anything, some standard or norm must be decided upon in order to make proper comparisons and in order to speak a common language with others. Since skulls and extracted teeth show so many variations and anomalies, an arbitrary norm for individual teeth had to be established for comparative study. It was thought that if the drawing and carving of the teeth would coincide with such an arbitrary norm as to measurements, one would ultimately be able to carve and articulate complete dental arches that might be used as a text in teaching. Each year when extracted teeth were sorted and dissected by students during the laboratory periods, a search was made for good specimens to be used for photographic study.

A camera was used to photograph the teeth, which allowed adjustment to take the photos exactly two diameters. The photographs of all aspects showed each tooth with its dimensions squared. These photographs were superimposed on squared millimeter cross section paper obtainable from engineers' supply firms. This procedure reduced the tooth outlines of each aspect to an accurate graph so that it was possible to compare and record the contours (Figs. 26, 27 and 28). (See pages 21 and 22).

Close observation of these outlines shows the relationship of crown to root, the extent of curvatures at various points, the inclination of roots, the relative widths of occlusal surfaces, the height of marginal ridges, contact areas, and so on.

Using the information obtained from the photographs, and through observation and calibration of thousands of teeth over a period of several years, dimensions were arbitrarily decided upon, and carvings were made

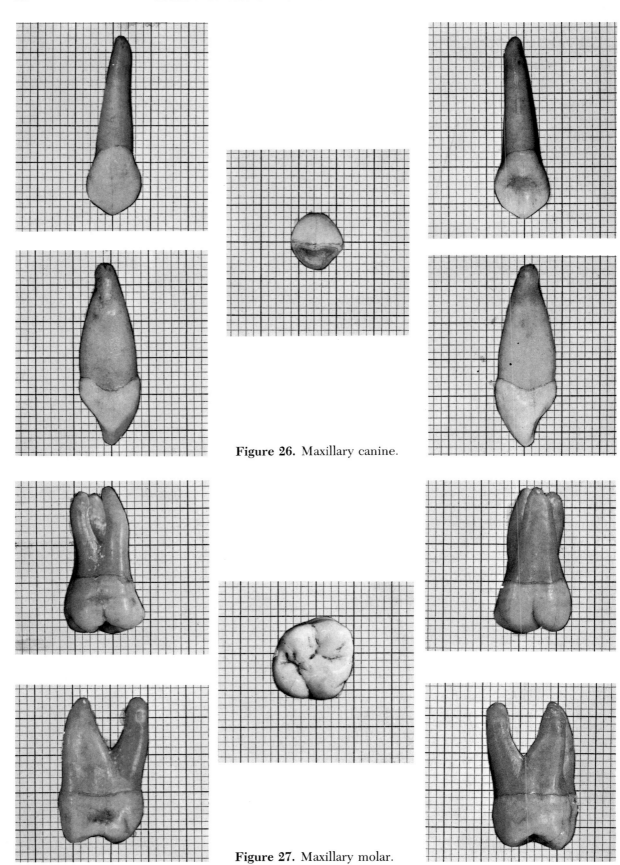

Figure 26. Maxillary canine.

Figure 27. Maxillary molar.

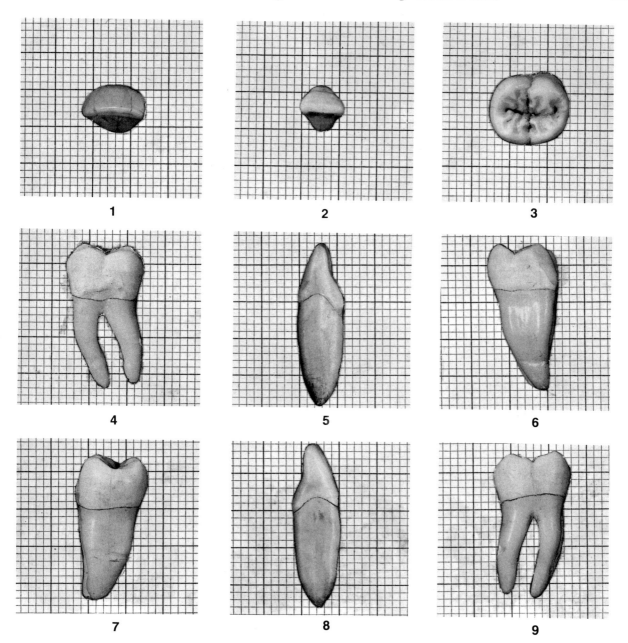

Figure 28. Actual photos of teeth raised to two diameters and superimposed on squared millimeters, reducing anatomic outlines to accurate graphs. *1*, Incisal aspect, maxillary central incisor; *2*, incisal aspect, mandibular lateral incisor; *3*, occlusal aspect, mandibular second molar; *4*, buccal aspect, mandibular second molar; *5*, mesial aspect, mandibular lateral incisor; *6*, mesial aspect, mandibular second molar; *7*, distal aspect, mandibular second molar; *8*, distal aspect, mandibular lateral incisor; *9*, lingual aspect, mandibular second molar.

in Ivorine. Then thirty-two teeth were carved, natural size, and placed in normal alignment and occlusion.

Although no claim is made that the table of measurements (page 26) established by the carvings is an average norm for tooth measurements, carvings and drawings made to those measurements will be generally accepted as approximately average.

The carvings in three dimensions, set up in normal alignment and occlusion, "proved" the table of measurements (Figs. 29, 30, and 131 A, B).

Calibrations in fractions of a millimeter were held to a minimum in simplifying the table. Necessary fractions are half millimeters (0.5), except for two instances where less than a half millimeter was required (refer to Table 1, page 26).

Fractions were avoided wherever possible in order to facilitate familiarity with the table and to avoid confusion. The student must memorize the table in order to be able to visualize tooth proportions instantly.

The table will assist students to carve with more ease than heretofore if they will calibrate their carvings accurately and adhere to the dimensions of their outlines. Accurate plans should be drawn of all the teeth, showing the five aspects as graphs on cross section paper and using the table of measurements as a basis. These drawings will assist the student by giving him conscious images in proportion. Carving in three dimensions later can then be accomplished more easily.

The successful student must be able to create accurate mental pictures

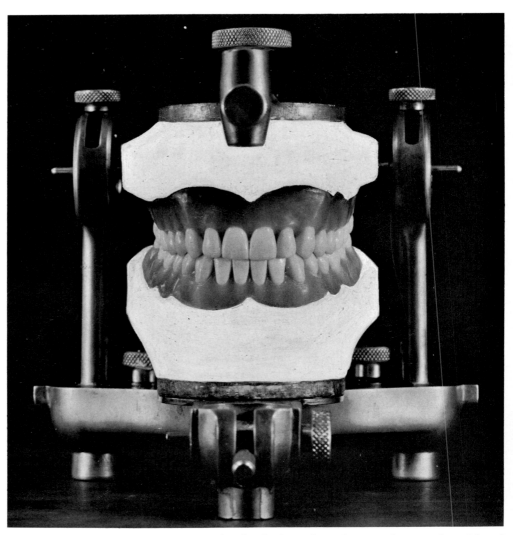

Figure 29. Carvings in Ivorine of individual teeth made according to the table of measurements on page 26. These models of teeth are set up into complete dental arches on an anatomic articulator.

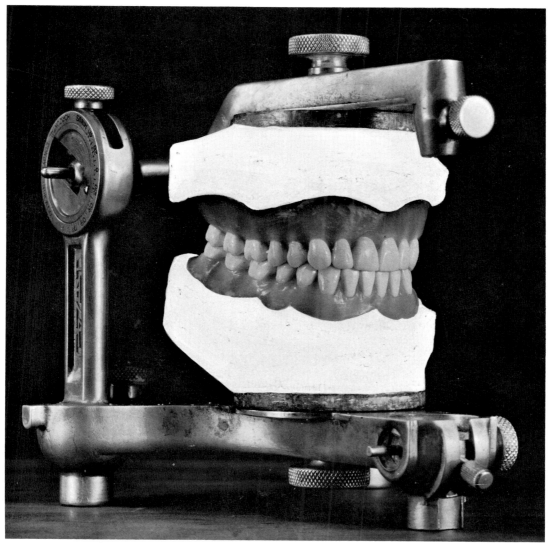

Figure 30. Another view of the model shown in Figure 29. See Figure 131, A and B, for enlarged occlusal views of these carvings.

of various aspects of the teeth. Complete pictures can be formed only when the individual is perfectly familiar with every detail—so familiar that it is possible for him to draw an outline of any aspect of any tooth in the human dental arches in good proportion without reference to a model. Then he should be capable of carving all or any part of a tooth to correspond to his drawings.

Acute observation comes only after habitual study of detail. With the necessary application and interest, any student can learn to be an authority on the anatomy of the teeth; and that is the first step in becoming a master operator.

Three main skills must be acquired for excellence.

1. Become so familiar with a table of measurements that it is possible to make instant comparisons mentally of the proportion of one tooth to another from any aspect.

2. Learn to draw accurate outlines of any aspect of any tooth.

3. Learn to carve with precision any design illustrated with line drawings.

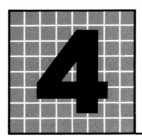

Plan for the Laboratory Course

Outline drawings of the five aspects of each tooth are to be completed first. They are drawn on graph paper according to the table of measurements.

Carving should not be attempted until the outline drawing of each aspect of each tooth to be carved is mastered (Fig. 46).

Carvings are then made of each tooth from blocks of plaster of Paris to the same scale as the drawings; ⅛ inch equals 1 millimeter. The method of accomplishing this will be described and illustrated in detail on following pages.

There is a good reason for beginners to start their elementary training with oversize drawings and carvings. The procedure is simplified visually for the student; the need for necessary corrections will be more apparent, whether noticed by the student himself or by an instructor.

Since graph paper scaled to ⅛ inch is available for drawing plans, the size of final plaster carvings is established. Carvings in that proportion will be *approximately three diameters*. Plaster carvings that are too large are not practical for many obvious reasons. Drawings and carvings three diameters are large enough for contrast; and the scale makes it convenient to use the one table of measurements for oversize plaster carvings first, and then make normal size carvings in millimeters later in some other medium.

The consensus among most instructors is that no more than eight plaster carvings are necessary. These will be the eight typical forms: central incisors, canines, first premolars and first molars, maxillary and mandibular (see Frontispiece).

After plaster carvings to three diameters are completed satisfactorily, sixteen *normal size* carvings to a millimeter scale are made in some other medium. These represent all the teeth of one side, including the third molars. Carving blocks may be obtained of hard carving wax, a plastic composition or bone. After all the individual carvings are completed, they are to be set up on an articulator (Figs. 105 to 108). Third molars are often omitted in the set-up because they are not usually included in prosthetic procedure.

Drawings and carvings of teeth portray an "ideal" or composite version of tooth outlines. For a more extensive study of dental anatomy showing actual photographs of typical specimens and variations, the reader is referred to the latest edition of *Dental Anatomy, Physiology* and *Occlusion*, W. B. Saunders Company.

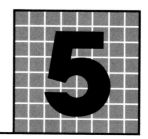

Drawing

Drawing the teeth is a help in learning details, but it is, of course, two dimensional only and is limited to fundamental outlines in the study of tooth form. It serves, however, to teach accuracy and to create mental pictures of proportion. From this we go to three-dimensional delineation, which is sculpture or carving.

Teeth are unique in that their outside form is functional; they are not capable of readaptation or of being rebuilt by the body in case of wear or accident. Therefore, those who are interested in the techniques of restorative dentistry must be able, through study and digital training, to restore form and function in the dental arches.

Outline drawings of each aspect of the tooth to be studied are made on graph paper. In order to standardize the technique further, the paper used has squares of sufficient size to make the drawings coincide with the size of the finished carvings in plaster of Paris to be made later. Models of this size are not unwieldy and yet are large enough to show detail whether they are used in the study of form or to show preparation design in operative or restorative procedure after the student advances to courses on dental technique.

Graph paper scaled to ⅛ inch is chosen (Fig. 46). The drawing scale of ⅛ inch = 1 millimeter results in drawings approximately three diameters in size.

Use of the above scale makes it easier for the student to mark off the various measurements when he is drawing outlines on plain paper or on the plaster blocks during carving technique. Six-inch rulers may be obtained with the inch scale on one edge and the metric scale on the other. Measuring off multiples of millimeters would be confusing and would multiply the chances of error.

The teeth are calibrated at certain points in accordance with the table of measurements. The dimensions of the maxillary central incisor are given as an example in Figure 31. The aspects to be drawn are incisal or occlusal, labial or buccal, lingual, mesial and distal. The five aspects may be drawn as graphs on one page with the incisal or occlusal view placed in the center (Figs. 46 and 48).

Table 1. Measurements of the Teeth (Millimeters) and Specifications for Drawing and Carving Teeth of Average Size

	Cervico-incisal Length of Crown	Length of Root	Mesio-distal Diameter of Crown	Mesio-distal Diameter at Cervix	Labio- or Bucco-lingual Diameter	Labio- or Bucco-lingual Diameter at Cervix	Curvature of Cervical Line— Mesial	Curvature of Cervical Line— Distal
Maxillary Teeth								
Central incisor	10.5	13.0	8.5	7.0	7.0	6.0	3.5	2.5
Lateral incisor	9.0	13.0	6.5	5.0	6.0	5.0	3.0	2.0
Canine (cuspid)	10.0	17.0	7.5	5.5	8.0	7.0	2.5	1.5
First premolar (bicuspid)	8.5	14.0	7.0	5.0	9.0	8.0	1.0	0.0
Second premolar (bicuspid)	8.5	14.0	7.0	5.0	9.0	8.0	1.0	0.0
First molar	7.0*	b 12 l 13	10.0	8.0	11.0	10.0	1.0	0.0
Second molar	6.5*	b 11 l 12	9.0	7.0	11.0	10.0	1.0	0.0
Third molar	6.0*	11.0	8.5	6.5	10.0	9.5	1.0	0.0
Mandibular Teeth								
Central incisor	9.0†	12.5	5.0	3.5	6.0	5.3	3.0	2.0
Lateral incisor	9.5†	14.0	5.5	4.0	6.5	5.8	3.0	2.0
Canine (cuspid)	11.0	16.0	7.0	5.5	7.5	7	2.5	1.0
First premolar (bicuspid)	8.5	14.0	7.0	5.0	7.5	6.5	1.0	0.0
Second premolar (bicupid)	8.0	14.5	7.0	5.0	8.0	7.0	1.0	0.0
First molar	7.5	14.0	11.0	9.0	10.5	9.0	1.0	0.0
Second molar	7.0	13.0	10.5	8.0	10.0	9.0	1.0	0.0
Third molar	7.0	11.0	10.0	7.5	9.5	9.0	1.0	0.0

The sum of the mesiodistal diameters, both right and left, which gives the arch length, is maxillary 128 mm., mandibular 126 mm.

*Buccal aspect.

†Lingual measurement approximately 0.5 mm. longer.

Close observation of the outline drawings on the squared background will show the relation of crowns to roots, extent of curvatures at various points, inclination of roots, relative widths of occlusal surfaces, height of marginal ridges, contact areas, etc.

Although there will be some description of each tooth, especially in drawing the "ideal" or "model" outlines in this atlas, more complete description with actual photographs of the teeth will be found in the textbook and may be studied along with the use of the atlas.

It is suggested that the student acquire a collection of tooth specimens of his own to be used in comparative study (Fig. 89).

Use of Measurement Table
In Outlining Drawings and Carvings
(measurements of the teeth in millimeters)

Maxillary Teeth	Cervico-Incisal Length of Crown	Length of Root	Mesio-Distal Diameter of Crown	Mesio-Distal Diameter of Crown at Cervix	Labio- or Bucco-Lingual Diameter of Crown	Labio- or Bucco-Lingual Diameter at Cervix	Curvature of Cervical Line—Mesial	Curvature of Cervical Line—Distal
Central Incisor	10.5	13.0	8.5	7.0	7.0	6.0	3.5	2.5

Sketches showing above dimensions as applied to
drawings or carvings checked with caliper

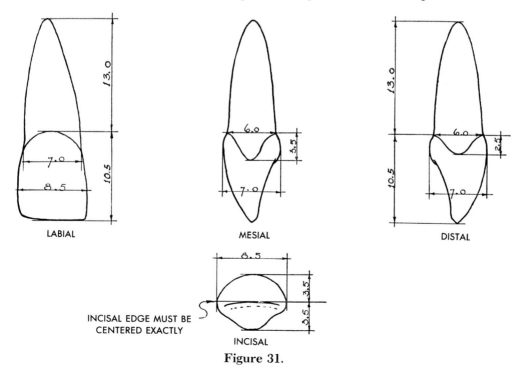

LABIAL   MESIAL   DISTAL

INCISAL EDGE MUST BE
CENTERED EXACTLY

INCISAL

Figure 31.

METHOD OF CALIBRATING AN ANTERIOR TOOTH

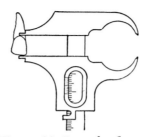

Figure 32. Length of crown.

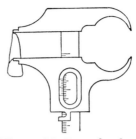

Figure 33. Length of root.

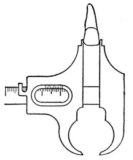

Figure 34. Mesiodistal diameter of crown.

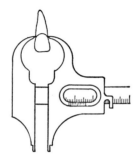

Figure 35. Mesiodistal diameter of crown at cervix.

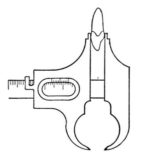

Figure 36. Labiolingual diameter of crown.

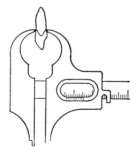

Figure 37. Labiolingual diameter of crown at cervix.

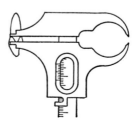

Figure 38. Curvature of cementoenamel junction on mesial.

METHOD OF CALIBRATING A POSTERIOR TOOTH

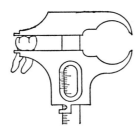

Figure 39. Length of crown.

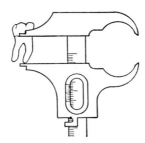

Figure 40. Length of root.

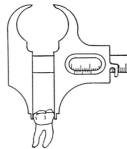

Figure 41. Mesiodistal di-ameter of crown.

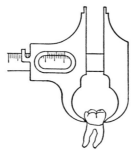

Figure 42. Mesiodistal di-ameter of crown at cervix.

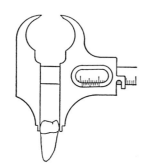

Figure 43. Buccolingual di-ameter of crown.

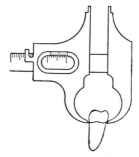

Figure 44. Buccolingual di-ameter of crown at cervix.

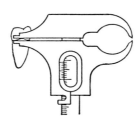

Figure 45. Curvature of cementoenamel junction on mesial.

MAXILLARY CANINE

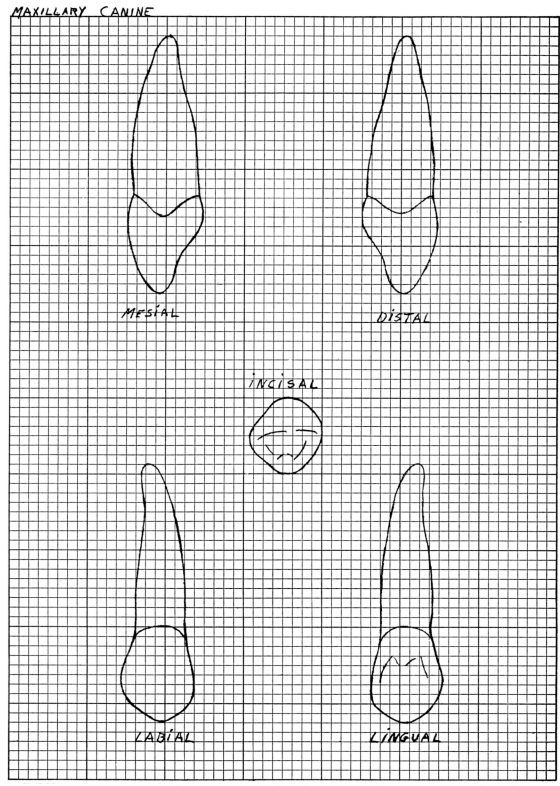

Figure 46. Graphs drawn in pencil as done by a student on engineers' graph paper scaled eight to the inch. Each square represents 1 millimeter in tooth measurement. Although the student did not make a perfect drawing and did not place aspects as suggested, the illustration serves its purpose. (Graph paper by Keuffel & Esser Co., N.Y., Catalogue #4, sheet #46–0622.)

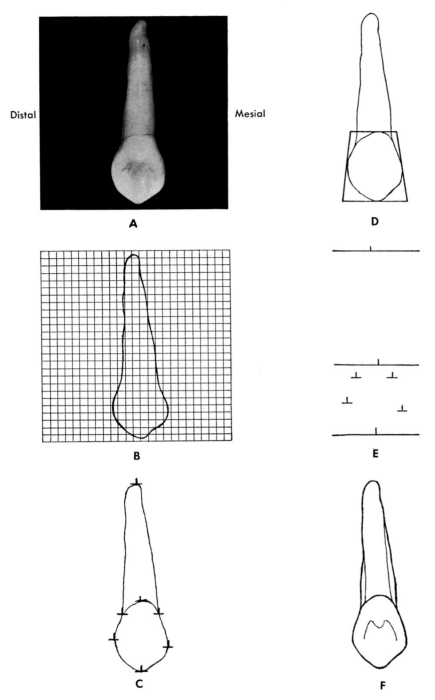

Distal   Mesial

A   D

B   E

C   F

Figure 47. Suggestions for practice in drawing outlines. Lingual aspect of the maxillary left canine. *A,* Photograph of natural tooth, representing a specimen used as a model; *B,* accurate graph of outline; *C,* points of calibration representing length of crown and root, crests of contour, cervical widths, etc.; *D,* drawing the crown form within a geometric figure sometimes helps as a suggestion of schematic form in freehand drawing in contrast to graph drawing; *E,* freehand drawing suggestion: lines and points are marked with pencil on paper or chalk on blackboard to represent dimensions and the points connected by outline drawing; *F,* example of freehand drawing of the tooth without the aid of graphs or point markings.

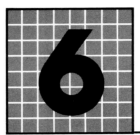

Individual Tooth Form, Maxillary Arch

The measurement of each tooth as found in the table on page 26 must be consulted before starting the drawing of the tooth in order to keep the proportions in mind. If the student is unfamiliar with the proportions, he cannot follow "a set of plans."

The various points in the description of individual teeth will be brought out by means of marginal sketches. This is the method of freehand drawing that should be practiced by students. After becoming thoroughly familiar with the measurements and after completing accurate graphs of the outlines of various aspects of any tooth on the graph paper, the student should practice freehand drawings, using only three horizontal lines for proportion, which lines represent the crown length and root length (Fig. 47 *E*).

MAXILLARY CENTRAL INCISOR

The maxillary central incisor, or first incisor, is the first tooth in the maxilla to the right or left of the median line (Fig. 48).

The crown length is as great as, or greater than, any of the other anterior teeth, *excepting the mandibular canine*, and its mesiodistal width is greater at the cervix and contact areas than in any other anterior tooth. Therefore, the area of the labial face of the crown of this tooth is greater in extent than any of the other anterior teeth.

The maxillary central incisors are the most prominent teeth and, therefore, the most noticeable in the dental arches. They are the most representative of the "mold design" of the teeth belonging to the individual, and together they form a focusing point for the eyes of observers.

This tooth has one well-developed root which is thick throughout with the apex bluntly rounded.

Labial Aspect

Lines are made representing the length of the crown cervicoincisally and the length of the root cervicoapically. The incisal edge will be placed at *a*, the crest of curve of the cervical line at *b*, and the apex of the root at *c*.

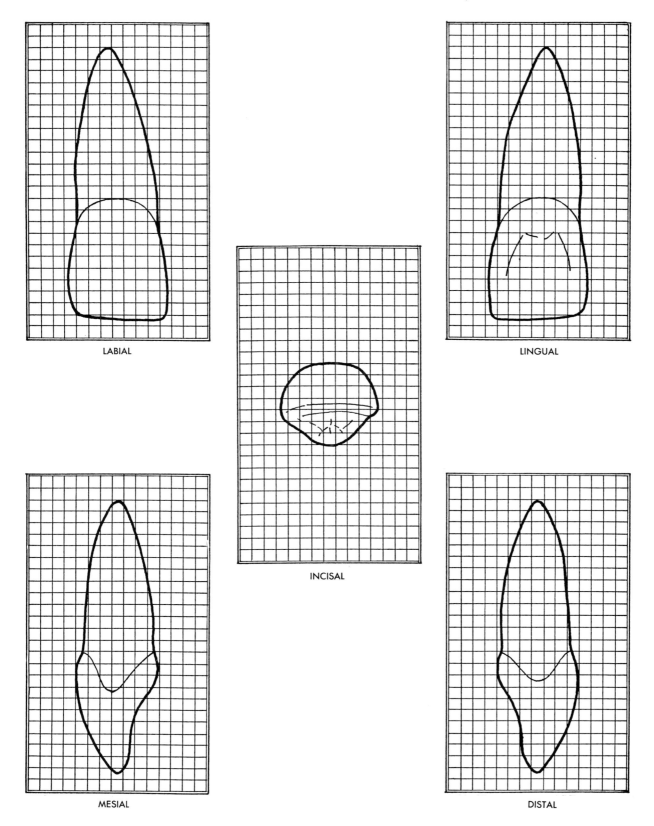

Figure 48. Maxillary right central incisor. In incisal view, labial aspect is at top of drawing.

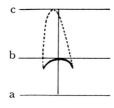

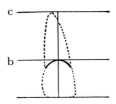

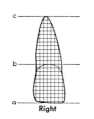

The cervical third of the crown is semi-elliptical in outline with the crest of curve at line *b*. The ends of the outline represent the approximate points at which the root outline joins the crown. The root is thick and cone-shaped with the apex of the cone rounded (dotted outline to line *c*).

The mesial outline of the crown is drawn next. From the point at which the root and crown join, the crown widens out mesially to make contact with the adjacent tooth, in this case the other central incisor. The mesioincisal angle of this incisor approaches a right angle in outline. Naturally, this form puts the contact with the other central incisor near the incisal edge.

The distal outline of the crown is more curved, with the crest of the curve closer to the middle third and the distoincisal angle much more rounded than the mesioincisal angle. The line *a* connects the mesial and distal outlines of the crown and completes the labial outline of the tooth.

The points at which the crests of the curve are placed on the mesial and distal are very important, since they represent the contact with the neighboring teeth. The slightest changes in the outlines will change the points of contact. The outline of the interproximal space will be changed at the same time and also the outline form of the incisal embrasures. (Make some sketches, changing the outlines, and note what happens to the embrasures and interproximal spaces.)

Lingual Aspect

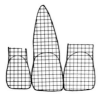

The lingual aspect may be outlined in the same manner as the labial aspect. The outstanding landmarks on the lingual side of the crown are the cingulum and the marginal ridges.

Mesial Aspect

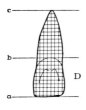

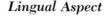

The mesial aspect brings out the form which classifies the central incisor as an incising instrument. The crown is wedge shaped, with its largest measurement at the crest of the curve labially and lingually, tapering down to the incisal edge.

A dotted line may be drawn bisecting lines *a*, *b*, *c*. This line represents the "axis" of the tooth. The line is to bisect the outline of the crown and root.

At about one-fifth the distance from *b* to *a*, two points are placed to represent the labiolingual crown measurement at the crests of curvature. Part of the labial outline of the crown is made by drawing a line almost straight but slightly convex, connecting the labial crest with the junction of the dotted line and *a*, which is the incisal edge.

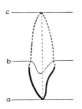

Part of the lingual outline is made by drawing a line concave and then convex from the crest of the curve to the incisal edge.

The labial and lingual outlines of the crown are completed by two short arcs connecting the two points representing the crest of curve labially and lingually with line *b* at the point of junction of crown and root. These two arcs represent a curve inward of approximately 0.5 mm. on each side. (Note in the measurement table the difference between the diameter of the crown labiolingually and the diameter at cervix labiolingually.)

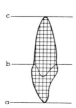

The root may be outlined as a blunt cone from the points at which the crown joins the root labially and lingually to the apex where the axis line bisects line *c*.

To complete the mesial aspect, the curvature of the cervical line on the mesial surface is outlined. It curves toward the incisal edge about one-third the length of the crown. The dotted line drawn through the center of the root and the center of the crown bisects the cervical curvature on the mesial and passes through the point outlined by the junction of the labial and lingual outlines at the incisal edge. This alignment is characteristic of maxillary central and lateral incisors. A straight line drawn through the root and crown of these teeth on the mesial or distal will rarely, if ever, pass through the lingual surface. Too often a drawing or carving of these teeth is made showing the crown off center to the labial.

Occasionally we find these teeth with the incisal edge to the lingual of center as in the so-called "hawk-bill" or "eagle-beak" incisor form.

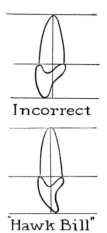

Incorrect

"Hawk Bill"

Distal Aspect

The distal aspect is practically a reverse outline to that of the mesial aspect. There is one important difference: the cervical curvature of the cementoenamel junction incisally is less in extent than that on the mesial surface. (Refer to the table of measurements.)

Incisal Aspect

As was mentioned, the incisal and occlusal aspects of the teeth are of the utmost importance in a study of dental anatomy. These views are the ones that teach proportion in crown outline form more than any other and show the relationship of the incisal edges and cusps to the bulk of the crown. In addition, outlines of these aspects of adjoining teeth in the arch, when placed together, will bring out contact design and embrasure form.

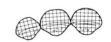

An outline of the maxillary central incisor from the incisal aspect should place the incisal edge directly in the center of the crown labiolingually.

Note the thickness of the crown at all points labiolingually. Without this thickness the proper contact and embrasure design would be impossible. Beginners are apt to design this crown too thin mesially and distally. Familiarity with the measurement table, together with proper observation of specimen teeth, will prevent such mistakes.

MAXILLARY LATERAL INCISOR

The maxillary lateral incisor, or second incisor, is the second tooth from the median line. This tooth resembles the central incisor in functional form. Although the dimensions of the crown are less in all directions, the root is usually just as long, but not so thick (Fig. 49). Since the lateral incisor is comparable in functional form, it helps to perform the same work in the mouth, namely, incision and apprehension of food.

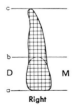

Right

The lateral incisor crown is likely to have the same typal form and outline as the central incisor of any given individual. However, there are many variations in this tooth. No other tooth in the mouth, except the third molar, is so apt to show odd forms. Anthropologists suggest that this tooth, like the third molar, is disappearing through the process of evolution, which would account for extreme variations, dwarfing, and frequent absence from the arch in the second dentition.

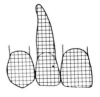

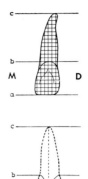

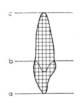

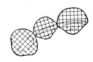

Dwarfed lateral incisors are not uncommon. They assume a tapered form at times, causing them to be dubbed "peg laterals." This anomaly is quite disfiguring to an otherwise normal mouth and necessitates esthetic restoration by the dentist.

The essential difference, aside from dimensions, between the outline form of the lateral incisor crown and that of the central incisor, from a labial view, is the rounded incisal edge and the level of the crest of curvature of the distal. The distal curvature in the lateral incisor places the contact area higher cervically than the contact area distal to the central incisor. Both mesial and distal "corners" are rounded. Therefore, the incisal outline from mesial contact area to distal contact area may be almost semicircular.

Great emphasis must be placed on contact areas and contact variations. In restorative procedures, the restoration of normal function of the teeth is the paramount consideration. No one detail in this work is more important than the restoration of proper contact form.

The root of the maxillary lateral incisor is rather round on cross section but slender lengthwise when compared with the central incisor. The root length is about the same but appears longer because the lateral crown is shorter than the central. The outline form of the root differs considerably because of the dimensions and the fact that it is usually curved somewhat near the apical end. It curves distally in most instances, but occasionally a curvature mesially may be seen in radiographs and specimens.

MAXILLARY CANINE*

The maxillary canine is the third tooth from the median line.

The canines are the only teeth with a single cusp and are so named because they reach their highest development in the carnivorous animals. (Latin *canis*—dog.)

The canine is a prehensile tooth; that is, its main function is the tearing and securing of food. Among the carnivora it is developed to the point of being useful in combat also.

The human canine when first erupted, before wear or abrasion has had a chance to change its appearance, looks very primitive, showing characteristics none of the other teeth possess. It has the longest and largest root of any tooth, a fact which assures its anchorage in the jaws. The canines are the longest teeth over-all in the mouth.

The crowns are beautifully designed for both strength and cleanliness under all stresses of wear and usage. Consequently, they are usually the last teeth to be lost, and often remain many years after the others are gone. These teeth, therefore, are most important as abutments in prosthetic restorations.

Because of their position in the arches and the length and angulation of the roots, all the canines act as important underlying structures of the face, assuring sufficient prominence at the "corners" of the mouth to bring out character, strength and beauty.

---

*The term *cuspid* is widely used in the United States only. Worldwide, the term *canine* is the one accepted by most scientific bodies interested in dental anatomy, human and comparative.

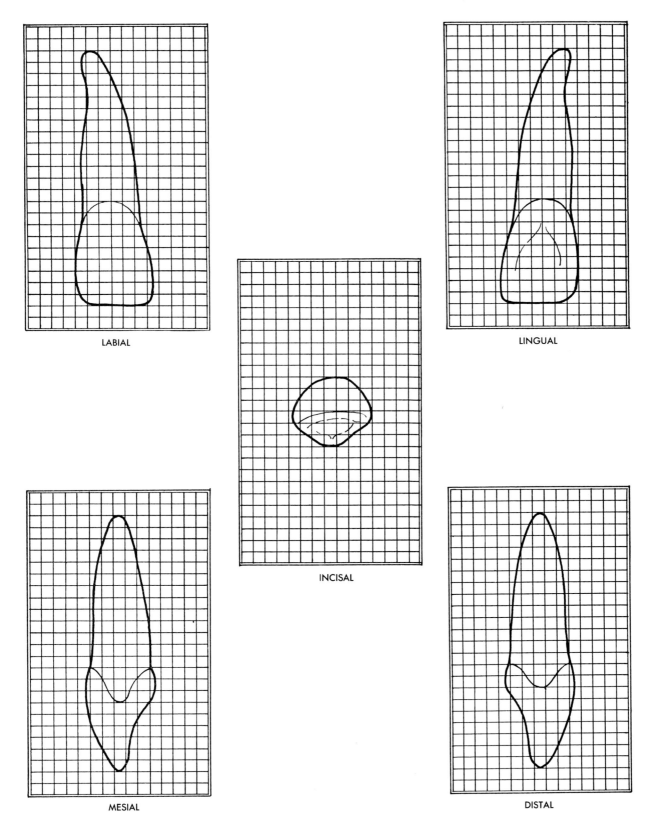

LABIAL

LINGUAL

INCISAL

MESIAL

DISTAL

Figure 49. Maxillary right lateral incisor.

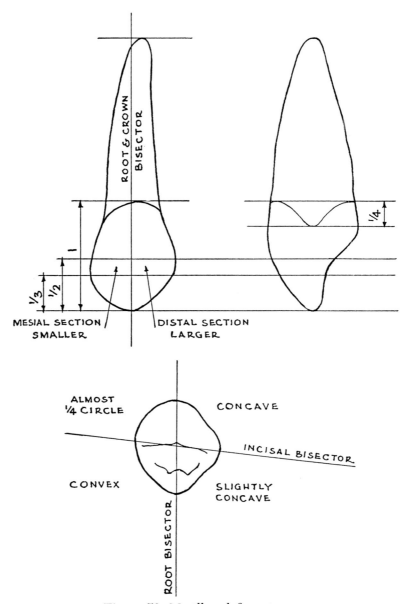

Figure 50. Maxillary left canine.

Labial Aspect

The cervical third of the maxillary canine crown is narrower than that of the central incisor because the root labially is slenderer. The root is long and tends to curve distally at the apex, tapering considerably. Although most roots curve more or less to the distal, this is not a hard and fast rule. A line drawn through the body of the crown and root of all teeth facially may show curvature to the distal, but many times a sharp curve to the mesial at the *apical third* will be found.

The *mesial outline of the crown* is convex, with the crest of the curvature at the junction of middle and incisal thirds of the crown, placing the contact with the lateral incisor in that location. The outline slants along the cusp to the cusp tip. The cusp tip will usually be bisected by the axis line through crown and root (Fig. 50).

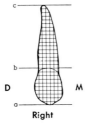

Right

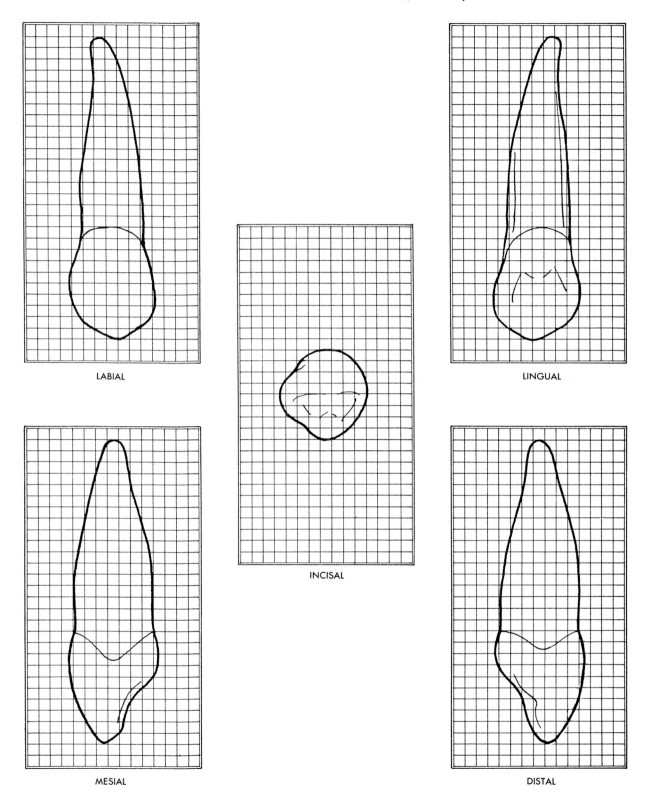

LABIAL

LINGUAL

INCISAL

MESIAL

DISTAL

Figure 51. Maxillary right canine.

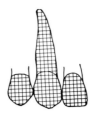

The *distal outline of the crown* is slightly concave from the junction of the crown and root to the distal contact area. This crest of curve is placed differently from the mesial crest; it is located at the center of the middle third of the crown. This point contacts the mesial surface of the first premolar.

To repeat, the contact area mesially is at the juncture of the middle and the incisal thirds; the contact area distally is at the middle third of the canine crown. Since the maxillary canine makes contact with the lateral incisor mesially and the first premolar distally (two dissimilar forms), the contact levels are adjusted accordingly. Physiologically, all the canines are anterior teeth mesially and posterior teeth distally (Fig. 50).

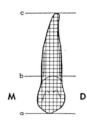

Lingual Aspect

The lingual aspect may be outlined as the reverse of the labial aspect. A natural tooth or a three dimensional model of one should be examined in order to study the form of the cingulum, the marginal ridges, and the way the transverse ridge merges with the tip of the cusp and the cingulum.

Mesial Aspect

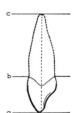

This aspect shows the canine to be functionally an incisor also because of its form. The crown is tapered from the crest of curvature labially and lingually down to the tip of the cusp, resembling the central and lateral incisors. The measurement labiolingually is greater than that of the central and lateral incisors, which gives the crown greater bulk and more reinforcement. In addition to the variance in dimensions, the pointed cusp form of the canine makes it deviate from the incisors.

At about *one-fourth* the distance from *b* to *a*, when one is drawing freehand,* two points are placed to represent the labiolingual crown measurement at the crests of curvature. Part of the labial outline of the crown is made by drawing a line almost straight, but slightly convex, connecting the labial crest with the tip of the cusp. You will notice that the tip of the cusp is not located on the axis line but is labial to it. This is characteristic of maxillary canines (Fig. 51).

Part of the lingual outline is made by drawing a line concave and then convex from the crest of the curve on the cingulum to the tip of the cusp.

The labial and lingual outlines are completed by two short arcs connecting the two points representing the crest of curve labially and lingually with line *b* at the point of junction of crown and root. These two areas represent a curve inward of approximately 0.5 mm. on each side, the same as found on maxillary central and lateral incisors.

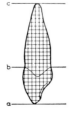

The root may be outlined as a rounded cone from the points at which the crown joins the root labially and lingually to the apex, where the axis line bisects line *c*. Often the apex of the root is found labial to this point.

To complete the mesial aspect, the curvature of the cementoenamel junction is outlined. It curves toward the incisal edge about one-fourth the length of the crown. (See measurement table, page 26, "Curvature of Cervical Line—Mesial.")

---

*It is suggested again that the student follow the text, making his own freehand drawings to correspond with the examples given as marginal drawings.

Distal Aspect

The distal aspect is a reverse outline to that of the mesial aspect. The line representing the curvature of cervical line on the distal surface differs, of course, being less in extent than that representing the curvature on the mesial surface.

Incisal Aspect

As illustrated in the accompanying marginal drawing, the canine outline is almost a series of arcs. The mesial surface from this aspect can be portrayed in a relatively long arc, the labial at the cervical third with a short one, the cingulum outline with another short arc, and the distal outline with another. The line representing the cusp with its incisal slopes is slightly labial to center, and the actual point of the cusp is placed so that a line bisecting the arcs labially and lingually will pass through it (Fig. 50).

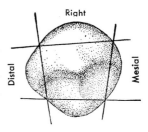

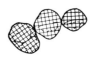

Note the greater diameter of the canine labiolingually. Also observe the concavity both labially and lingually toward the distal where the distal arc joins the labial and lingual arcs.

MAXILLARY FIRST PREMOLAR*

The maxillary first premolar is the fourth tooth from the median line in the maxilla. Premolars and molars are called posterior teeth; therefore, the first premolar is the first posterior tooth distal to the median line.

This tooth has two cusps, one buccal and one lingual, giving rise to the term bicuspid, a term widely used by dentists in the United States. However, because the mandibular first premolar has only one functioning cusp and the second mandibular premolar has three on the average, the term bicuspid is not generally acceptable.

This tooth often has two separate well-formed roots, a buccal root and a lingual root. The bifurcation often occurs at the middle third of the root. It is this type which will be drawn as average.

Often the tooth will appear with one root only, but this root will contain two pulp canals.

Buccal Aspect

The line describing the cementoenamel junction on the buccal surface curves less than those describing any of the anterior teeth. The reason for this is that the curvature of the cementoenamel junction on the mesial and distal is less; therefore, the continuation describing the curvature buccally is less.

The *root* is much shorter than the canine root but, aside from the dimensions, the outline from the buccal aspect resembles the labial aspect of the canine root. The apical third is slenderer, with a finer taper at the

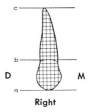

---

*Since the term *premolar* is the one which is accepted by odontologists and the majority of scientific bodies interested in dental anatomy, human and comparative, it is the term which will be given preference here.

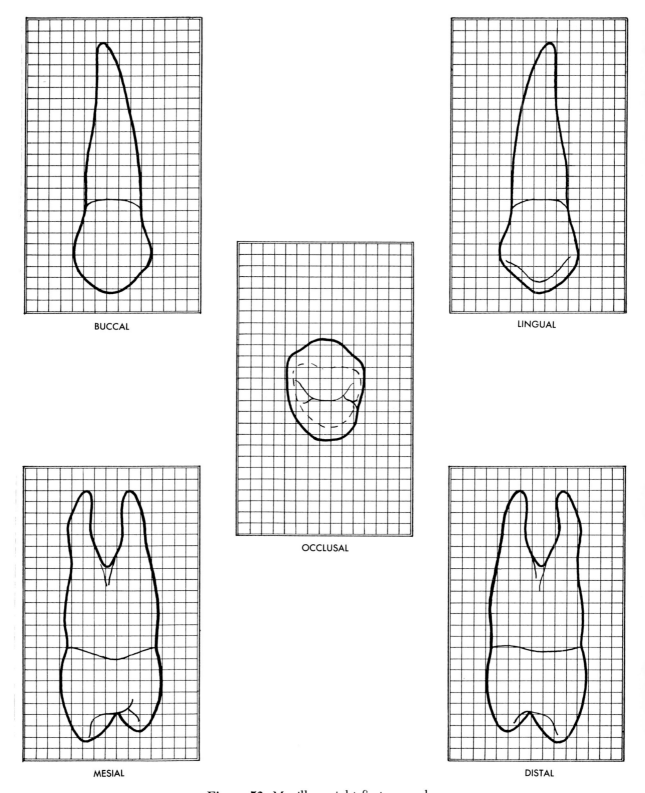

BUCCAL

LINGUAL

OCCLUSAL

MESIAL

DISTAL

Figure 52. Maxillary right first premolar.

apex. The mesial outline of the root is generally convex, with a distal concavity at the middle and apical thirds.

The *mesial outline of the crown* is concave above the contact area. The outline at the contact area is convex. The line progresses from this area to the tip of the buccal cusp with a slight indentation.

The *distal outline of the crown* is almost a straight line from the junction of crown and root to the contact area. The curved line from this point to the tip of the cusp is convex, differing from the slope to the mesial.

A line bisecting the contact areas at the crest of curvature will be slightly more than half the distance from cervical line to the tip of the cusp. This is characteristic of all the posterior teeth.

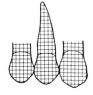

Lingual Aspect

The lingual aspect presents the same outline, with the addition of a curved line portraying the lingual cusp about 1 mm. shorter than the buccal cusp.

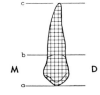

Mesial Aspect

Here one comes to the design which shows a characteristic of all maxillary posterior teeth. *The tips of the cusps are well within the confines of the root base, with the distance from cusp tip to cusp tip little more than half that of the calibration at the buccal and lingual crests of curvature of the crown. This characteristic proportion is true of all the posterior teeth, maxillary and mandibular* (Figs. 52, 53 and 54).

The measurement of the crown of the maxillary first premolar buccolingually at its greatest curvature compared with the measurement from buccal cusp tip to lingual cusp tip has been drawn in this manual in the ratio of 9 mm. to 5 mm. The ratio of 9 to 5 is typical of the proportion of those measurements in all posterior teeth, maxillary and mandibular. This fundamental ratio is most important in the study of tooth form and must be remembered. If the student keeps this ratio in mind, his drawings and carvings (and restorations later in operative procedure) should be in proportion, in this respect, within a fraction of a millimeter. As an example, when carving a molar with a buccolingual measurement of 12 mm., five-ninths of 12 would be 6⅔ or approximately 6.7 mm. If the calibration from cusp tip to cusp tip buccolingually is carved to measure anywhere from 6 mm. to 7 mm., the carving would still be correct within a fraction of a millimeter and would be in good proportion.

At about one-third the distance from *b* to *a* (Fig. 53), two points are placed to represent the buccolingual crown measurement at the crests of curvature. A point is placed on line *a*, one-third the measurement between those points, to locate the tip of the buccal cusp. Another dot is placed slightly above line *a* to denote the tip of the lingual cusp, allowing a little more than half the buccolingual measurement of the crown between the two cusp markings.

Part of the buccal outline of the crown is made by drawing a line slightly convex from the point representing the buccal crest to the tip of the buccal cusp. A similar line is drawn from the lingual crest to the tip of the lingual cusp. Now continue the outline from the tips of the cusps to a point half the distance between the cusp tips and a little more than one-fourth

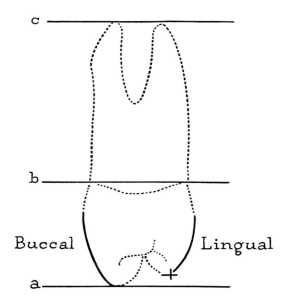

Figure 53. Maxillary right first premolar, mesial aspect.

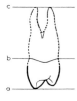

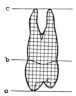

the distance from *a* to *b*. This outline brings out the slope between the cusps on the occlusal surface of the crown ending in the central groove.

A line is now drawn to mark the mesial marginal ridge with an extension on it to show a well-defined developmental groove which is characteristic of this tooth on the mesial surface.

The buccal and lingual outlines of the crown are completed by two short arcs connecting the two points at the crest of curvature buccally and lingually with line *b* at the point of junction with crown and root.

These continuations represent a curve inward the same as that found on centrals, laterals and canines. In fact, all the maxillary teeth will have about the same curvature at this point, approximately 0.5 mm. on each side. (Check graph drawings.)

The root may be outlined to show bifurcation for about half its length. Both root tips come to a rather fine taper, and each tip tends to be in line with the tip of its respective cusp—buccal or lingual.

To complete the mesial aspect, the cervical curvature of the cementoenamel junction is drawn. It curves only slightly toward the occlusal surface of the crown, approximately 1 mm.

Distal Aspect

The distal aspect presents the same outline as the mesial, with the lingual and buccal on opposite sides. The completed drawing shows less curvature of the cervical line and no developmental groove crossing the marginal ridge.

Although small developmental grooves may appear on any of the marginal ridges on any of the maxillary posterior teeth, they are so small that only the definite one to the mesial of the first premolar will be considered as significant or characteristic.

Occlusal Aspect

The salient points to be brought out on the drawing of this aspect are the relative positions of the contact areas and the relationship of the cusps

Figure 54. Maxillary right first premolar.

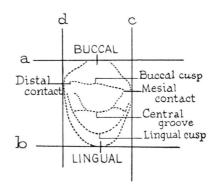

and central groove to the outline. Also to be remembered is the comparison between the mesiodistal width of the crown toward the buccal and the mesiodistal width toward the lingual (Fig. 131 A).

Mark off a rectangle with lines *a* and *b*, *c* and *d* (Fig. 54). The measurement between *a* and *b* will represent the width of the crown buccolingually, and the distance between *c* and *d* will represent the width mesiodistally.

Now put in four short crosslines—two to represent the crests of curvature at the contact area, mesial and distal, and the other two to represent the crests of curvature at the buccal surface and at the lingual surface. You will note that the point of greatest curvature of the buccal surface is about half the distance from *c* to *d*, and the highest point of curvature on the lingual surface is a little to the mesial of center; also that the center of the mesial contact area is about one-third the distance from *a* to *b*, and that of the distal contact area is about one-fourth the distance from *a* to *b*.

Practice completing the outline according to the illustration of the graph of this aspect.

It should be noted, in addition, that the line of the central groove on the occlusal surface with its supplementary grooves extending into the triangular fossae is nearer to the lingual outline than to the buccal outline.

The dotted lines representing the tips of the cusps and the crest of the marginal ridges show the buccal cusp to be farther from the buccal outline than the lingual cusp is from the lingual outline, and also that the crests of the marginal ridges are well within the outline of the contact areas. Check these points on the drawings of the other aspects or, better still, observe closely a good natural specimen of this tooth.

MAXILLARY SECOND PREMOLAR

The maxillary second premolar is the fifth tooth from the median line in the maxilla. Since this tooth supplements the first premolar in function, the outline form of all the aspects is similar.

Compare the graphs in Figure 55 with those in Figure 52, observing the following variations:

The second maxillary premolar is less angular. The sulcus on the occlusal surface between the cusps is more shallow, making the cusps shorter in relation to it. The occlusal surface of the maxillary second premolar is not so smooth as that of the first, presenting more of a "wrinkled" appearance (Fig. 131 A).

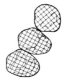

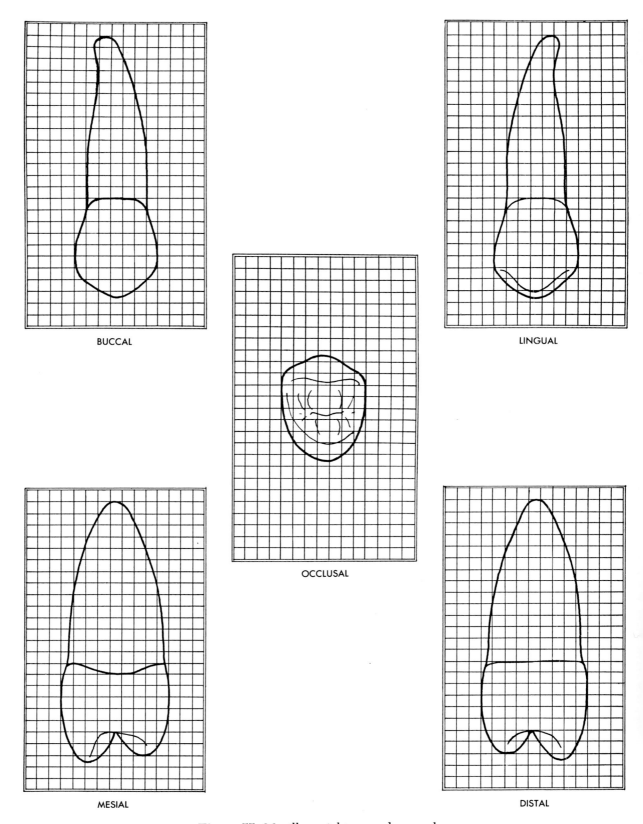

BUCCAL

LINGUAL

OCCLUSAL

MESIAL

DISTAL

Figure 55. Maxillary right second premolar.

The lingual cusp is nearly as long as the buccal cusp. Sometimes it is the same length.

There are more supplementary grooves on the occlusal surface, with a shorter central developmental groove.

There is no marked developmental groove in the mesial marginal ridge. In order to distinguish between right and left maxillary premolars, check the position of the contact areas mesially and distally. The mesial contact area will approach the center of the crown buccolingually and the distal contact area will be more off-center and toward the buccal surface (Figs. 54 and 55).

The tooth usually has one root, which presents a blunt cone outline from the mesial and distal aspects.

MAXILLARY FIRST MOLAR

The maxillary first molar is the sixth tooth from the median line in the maxilla. Normally it is the largest tooth in the maxillary arch. It has four well-developed cusps and one supplemental cusp called a fifth cusp or the cusp of Carabelli. The latter cusp is found to the lingual of the mesiolingual cusp, which is the largest of the well-developed ones. Quite often the fifth cusp is so poorly developed that it is hardly distinguishable. On close inspection, however, a developmental groove will always be found (unless erased by frictional wear) to show traces of cusp development at the usual site. This anatomic characteristic identifies the maxillary first molar.

Normally the tooth will have three well-developed roots, well separated.

The names of anatomical landmarks will be found in Figures 56, 57, and 58.

Buccal Aspect

The line describing the cementoenamel junction on the buccal surface is almost straight, dipping slightly as it joins the mesial and distal outline of the crown to denote a slight curvature of the cementoenamel junction mesially and distally on the crown (Fig. 59).

The *mesial outline of the crown* is very slightly concave above the contact area. The continuation of the line describing the contact area is convex and relatively broad, with its crest of curvature in the middle third of the crown near the junction of occlusal and middle thirds. The line progresses from this area to the tip of the mesiobuccal cusp with the line still convex.

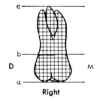

Right

Figure 56. Maxillary right first molar—occlusal landmarks. *MBCR*, Mesiobuccal cusp ridge; *CF*, central fossa (shaded area); *MTF*, mesial triangular fossa (shaded area); *MMR*, mesial marginal ridge; *MLCR*, mesiolingual cusp ridge; *OR*, oblique ridge; *DLCR*, distolingual cusp ridge; *DF*, distal fossa; *DTF*, distal triangular fossa (shaded area); *DMR*, distal marginal ridge; *DBCR*, distobuccal cusp ridge.

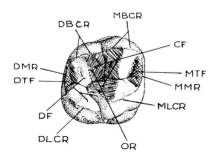

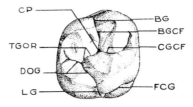

Figure 57. Maxillary right first molar—occlusal aspect—developmental grooves. *BG,* Buccal groove; *BGCF,* buccal groove of central fossa; *CGCF,* central groove of central fossa; *FCG,* fifth cusp groove; *LG,* lingual groove; *DOG,* distal oblique groove; *TGOR,* transverse groove of oblique ridge; *CP,* central pit.

Figure 58. Maxillary right first molar—buccal aspect. *DBR,* Distobuccal root; *LR,* lingual root; *MBR,* mesiobuccal root; *CL,* cervical line; *DBC,* distobuccal cusp; *MLC,* mesiolingual cusp; *BDG,* buccal developmental groove; *MBC,* mesiobuccal cusp.

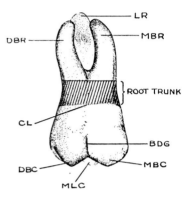

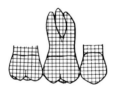

The *distal outline of the crown* is convex throughout. The crest of curvature which centers the contact area is closer to the center of the middle third of the crown than is the contact to the mesial.

Most of the distal surface of the crown may be seen from this aspect; therefore, the distobuccal cusp should be drawn to show traces of the distal marginal ridge. Two short lines, straight or slightly concave, are drawn to complete the outline of the buccal cusps, joining the lines extending from the cusp tips at the buccal groove in the center of the crown mesiodistally.

The length of cusps at this point will represent about 20 per cent of the total length of the crown. The mesiobuccal cusp will show greater width mesiodistally than the distobuccal cusp.

To complete the buccal aspect of the drawing from this angle, the mesiolingual cusp must show between the bifurcation of the two buccal cusps.

All *three* of the *roots* are in view from this aspect—two buccal roots and one lingual root. The *mesial outline* of the *mesiobuccal root* is concave above the cementoenamel junction for about one-third of its length. The outline curves to the mesial through the middle third, then curves sharply to the distal for the remainder of the apical third, ending in a taper slightly distal to a line bisecting the mesiobuccal cusp.

The *distal outline* of the *distobuccal root* is also concave at the cervical third above the cementoenamel junction of the middle third of the mesial root. Then the outline curves to the distal at the middle third, coming approximately to a level with the cementoenamel junction of the crown to the distal. The outline continues by curving to the mesial, ending in a tapered apex of the distal root just about on a line with the distobuccal cusp of the crown.

The distal outline of the mesiobuccal root and the mesial outline of the distobuccal root are portrayed by two concave lines connecting the apices of both roots with the point of their bifurcation, which is directly above the center of the crown buccally a little less than half their total length. A groove leading up to the actual bifurcation from below the junction of cervical and middle thirds should be indicated.

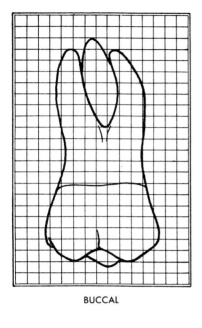

BUCCAL

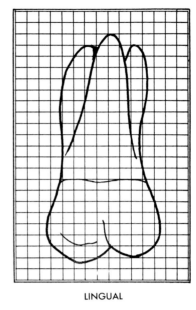

LINGUAL

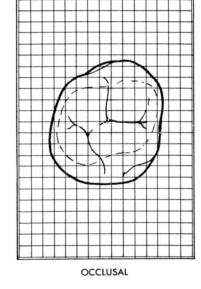

OCCLUSAL

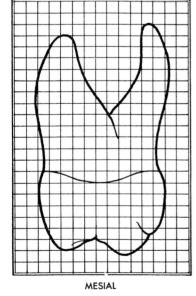

MESIAL

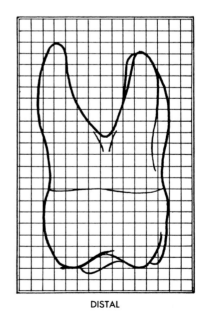

DISTAL

Figure 59. Maxillary right first molar.

The *lingual root* should be drawn immediately opposite the bifurcation from this aspect and somewhat longer than the buccal roots, usually about 1 mm.

Lingual Aspect

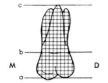

The line describing the cementoenamel junction of the crown is almost straight, often dipping slightly toward the occlusal and ending, of course, in a slight curve both mesial and distal as it joins the outline of the crown.

The mesial and distal outlines of the crown through the contact areas do not differ from the buccal aspects. The cusp outlines, however, are different.

The mesiolingual cusp is longer by about 0.5 mm. than any of the other cusps and, in addition, it is wider mesiodistally than any of the others.

The distolingual cusp is semicircular in outline from the point at which it joins the contact area to the lingual groove, which groove seems to continue the circular design, coming to rest at a point almost in the center of the crown mesiodistally and cervico-occlusally. The distolingual cusp is definitely shorter than the mesiolingual. The sulcus between the cusps is distal to the center of the crown outline.

To complete the drawing of the lingual aspect, a curved line is drawn directly above the mesiolingual cusp tip about 1.5 mm., outlining the position of the fifth cusp.

The *root outlines* of the buccal roots as shown from this aspect are repetitions of those just described for the buccal aspect, except, of course, that the mesial and distal outlines of the tooth from this aspect are reversed.

The *lingual root* must be drawn its entire length from this aspect, completely obliterating the outline of the space between the buccal roots. The lingual root is very wide at its base, the outline of it starting in the cervical third from this angle both mesial and distal, just inside the outline of the mesial and distal roots. The root is bluntly cone shaped and very regular in outline, slightly longer than the buccal roots and much stronger and heavier than either of them.

Mesial Aspect

The cervical line has a curvature toward the occlusal of about 1 mm. Sometimes it is less.

The *buccal outline of the crown* curves outward from the cementoenamel junction about 0.5 mm. (the same curvature as found on *all* maxillary teeth) to a point a little less than one-third the length of the buccal cusp, then continues the convexity to the tip of the cusp which is on a line with the apex of the mesiobuccal root.

The *lingual outline of the crown* describes the same extent of curvature from the cervical line to the crest of curvature on the lingual, then continues its convexity to complete the fifth cusp in line with the apex of the lingual root.

The *fifth cusp* in most instances is not a distinct cusp but a projection separated from the mesiolingual cusp by a developmental groove. Since this cusp arrangement is the most common it is the one described.

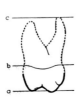

The *mesiolingual cusp* is outlined on the lingual from the developmental groove of the fifth cusp to its apex, which is in line with a point slightly lingual to the bifurcation of the roots.

The occlusal outline from this aspect is completed by drawing the outline of the mesial marginal ridge which dips toward the cervix from the tips of the cusps a little more than 1 mm., as a rule.

The same proportional relationship is present in the molars as was found in premolars; namely, *the distance from cusp tip to cusp tip buccolingually is a little better than one-half the total measurement of the calibration made at the crests of curvature of the crown buccolingually.*

The buccal outline of the mesiobuccal root is slightly concave above the cervical line, then bows out to a level even with or slightly buccal to the crest of the crown outline at the middle third of the root, then curves inward to end in a rounded apex directly in line with the mesiobuccal cusp of the crown.

The lingual outline of the lingual root is more concave above the cervical line than the buccal root; it continues on with a convex outline to a point above the middle third of the root and to a point lingual to the greatest curvature of the crown, then turns sharply inward to end in a tapered apex directly in line with the fifth cusp of the crown.

The drawing of the roots is completed by two concave lines drawn from the apices of the roots to the point of bifurcation a little to the lingual of the center of the drawing buccolingually and a little below the halfway point on the buccal root apices cervically. The lingual line describing the mesiobuccal root is continued to a point below the bifurcation and two-thirds the distance from the buccal outline of the buccal root to the lingual outline of the lingual root. This extension shows the starting point of the bifurcation mesially.

The *distobuccal root* is completely hidden from this aspect by the width of the mesiobuccal root buccolingually.

Distal Aspect

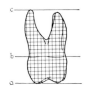

Because the maxillary first molar has considerable breadth and thickness, the drawing of this view is complicated by the rules of perspective. Therefore, it will be impossible to outline the drawing of the distal aspect correctly within the confines of a tracing of the mesial aspect.

A study of the drawing of the distal aspect will emphasize certain details which make it differ from the mesial aspect.

The line describing the cementoenamel junction on the distal surface is nearly straight, showing very little curvature.

Because of the slope on the buccal surface of the crown (see illustration of occlusal aspect), part of the mesiobuccal cusp may be seen beyond the distobuccal cusp.

The tip of the distobuccal cusp is in line with the apex of the distobuccal root.*

Part of the mesiolingual cusp is in view beyond the distal marginal ridge.

The distobuccal root is in full view, superimposed over the mesiobuccal root.

The distobuccal root is more slender in its entirety than the mesiobuccal root.

---

*Although it is not uncommon to find maxillary first molars with the distobuccal cusp overdeveloped, making it somewhat longer than the mesiobuccal cusp, usually this is not the case. The position of this tooth in the jaw causes the distobuccal cusp to appear longest because the roots are tipped distally and buccally, dropping the distobuccal cusp below the level of the mesiobuccal cusp (Fig. 138).

The point at which the distobuccal and lingual roots bifurcate is more nearly centered over the crown portion of the tooth.

Occlusal Aspect

The points to be brought out on the drawing of this aspect are the relative positions of the contact areas, the relationship of the cusps to each other, the design of the grooves on the occlusal surfaces, the width of the crown buccolingually as compared to mesiodistally, and the rhomboidal outline of the crown generally.

A good way to study the design of the occlusal aspect is to draw a rectangle on a piece of tracing paper with the same length and breadth as the crown measurements buccolingually and mesiodistally; place this over the illustration and check the salient points with the geometric figure as a contrast (Fig. 60).

This procedure may be adapted to any of the illustrations of crown form or root form wherever desired. Some students are able to get a clearer mental picture this way than by studying the graphs.

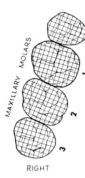

MAXILLARY MOLARS

RIGHT

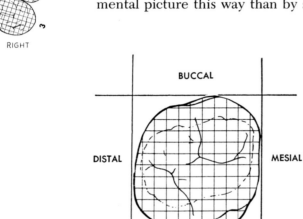

BUCCAL

DISTAL   MESIAL

LINGUAL

Figure 60. Maxillary right first molar, occlusal aspect.

MAXILLARY SECOND MOLAR

The maxillary second molar is the seventh maxillary tooth from the median line. Because it supplements the first molar in function, the design is similar. Compare the graphs of the second molar, Figure 61, with those of the first molar, Figure 59, observing the following variations:

Buccal Aspect

The crown is shorter cervico-occlusally and narrower mesiodistally.

The distobuccal cusp shows less development, allowing more of the distal marginal ridge and part of the distolingual cusp to be seen.

The roots are about the same length, but give the impression of being longer because the crown is shorter and the roots are closer together at the apices with their axes more nearly parallel.

The roots are inclined distally at a more extreme angle, placing the crest of curvature distally of the distobuccal root slightly distal to the distal extremity of the crown. The apex of the mesiobuccal root, by the same token, is on a line with the buccal groove of the crown instead of the tip of the mesiobuccal cusp as found on the first molar.

Lingual Aspect

The differences to be noted here in addition to those mentioned above are these:

The distolingual cusp of the crown is smaller.

The distobuccal cusp may be seen through the sulcus between the mesiolingual and distolingual cusps.

There is no fifth cusp.

The apex of the lingual root is in line with the distolingual cusp tip instead of the lingual groove.

Mesial Aspect

The buccolingual diameter of the crown is about the same; crown length is less.

The fifth cusp is missing.

The roots do not spread so far buccolingually, being within the confines of the buccolingual crown calibration.

Distal Aspect

Because of the angulation of the buccal surface, the mesiobuccal cusp may be seen from this angle.

The mesiolingual cusp cannot be seen.

The apex of the lingual root is inside a line bisecting the distolingual cusp.

Occlusal Aspect

The buccolingual diameter of the crown is about the same as that of the first molar, but the mesiodistal diameter is less.

The mesiobuccal and mesiolingual cusps are just as large and well developed, but the distobuccal and distolingual cusps are smaller and less well developed.

The measurement of the crown at the greatest diameter buccal and lingual to the distal cusps is considerably less than one made at the greatest diameter buccal and lingual to the mesial cusps; from the occlusal aspect, the crown tapers more distally than that of the first molar.

There is no fifth cusp.

The general shape of the occlusal aspect is also rhomboidal in character but with more extreme angulation than that of the maxillary first molar.

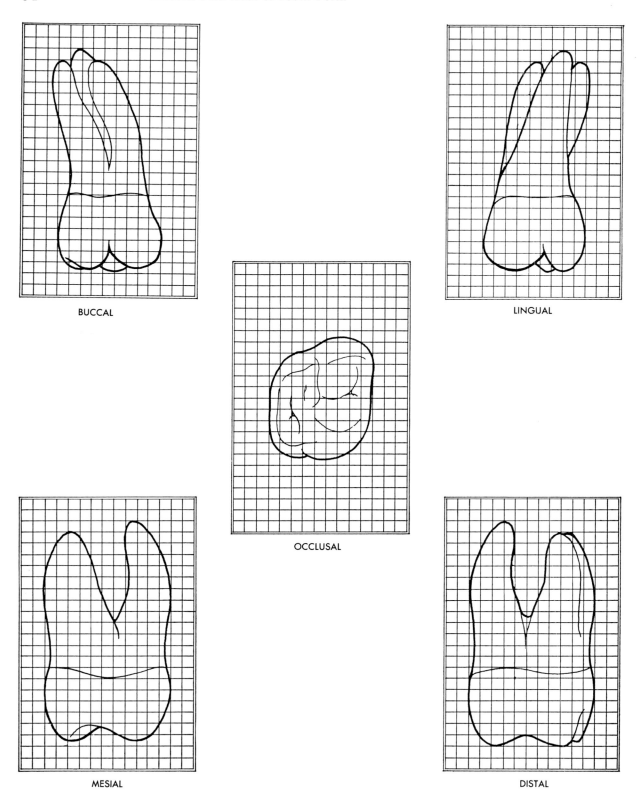

BUCCAL

LINGUAL

OCCLUSAL

MESIAL

DISTAL

Figure 61. Maxillary right second molar.

MAXILLARY THIRD MOLAR

The maxillary third molar is the eighth and last maxillary tooth from the median line. Because it supplements the second molar in function the fundamental design is similar. The tooth is smaller and not so well developed.

This tooth shows many variations in different individuals, but for the purposes at hand the illustrations will demonstrate a composite or average third molar. Actually, third molars may assume many malformations.

In making comparisons with the second molar the following points should be observed.

Buccal Aspect

The crown is shorter cervico-occlusally and narrower mesiodistally.

The roots are fused together, functioning as one large root, and are shorter cervicoapically.

The fused roots end in a taper at the apex.

The mesial outline of the roots has a more extreme slant to the distal, giving the apices of the fused roots a more distal relationship to the center of the crown.

Lingual Aspect

In addition to the differences mentioned above, there is just one large lingual cusp and, therefore, no lingual groove.*

Mesial Aspect

Here, aside from the differences in measurements as noted, the main feature is the taper to the fused roots and a bifurcation in evidence in the region of the apical third.

Distal Aspect

From this aspect most of the buccal surface of the crown is in view.

Part of the occlusal surface may be seen because of the angulation of the occlusal surface in relation to the long axis (see Buccal Aspect).

The measurement from the cervical line to the marginal ridge is short.

Occlusal Aspect

The occlusal aspect presents a heart-shaped outline (Fig. 62).

The lingual cusp is large and well developed.

---

*In many cases, third molars with the same essential features will present a small, poorly developed distolingual cusp with a developmental groove lingually.

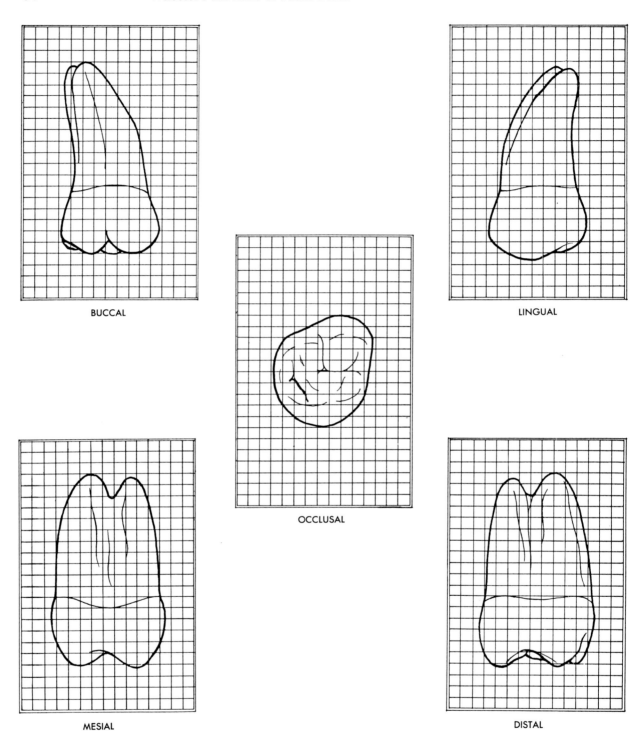

BUCCAL

LINGUAL

OCCLUSAL

MESIAL

DISTAL

Figure 62. Maxillary right third molar.

There is no distolingual cusp.* The tooth has a semicircular outline from one contact area to the other.

Only three cusps are shown.

---

*In many cases, third molars with the same essential features will present a small, poorly developed distolingual cusp with a developmental groove lingually.

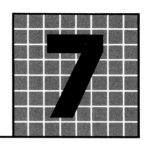

Individual Tooth Form, Mandibular Arch

MANDIBULAR CENTRAL INCISOR

The mandibular central or first incisor is the first tooth in the mandible right or left of the median line.

This tooth is the smallest one in the dental arches. The crown has little more than half the mesiodistal diameter of the maxillary central incisor. However, *the labiolingual diameter at its greatest calibration is only about 1 mm. less than that of the maxillary central incisor.* This is an important item to be considered when either the mandibular central or lateral incisors are involved in operative or restorative procedures. *The bulk in a labiolingual direction will discount to some extent the difficulties prompted by the tiny mesiodistal diameter.*

Restoration of the crown of this tooth and that of the lateral incisor requires the utmost skill because of the delicacy of their contours. *Advantage must be taken of their bulk labiolingually.* Fortunately, the mandibular incisors do not require treatment so often as other teeth, but they will need it often enough to test the art and skill of those responsible for restoration.

The single root is very narrow mesiodistally, although the root length is about the same as that of the maxillary central incisor.

Labial Aspect

The labial aspect is very regular and simple in outline, tapering evenly from the mesio- and distoincisal angles to the apex of the root.

The line describing the incisal edge of the crown is straight, with the mesioincisal angle sharp and the distoincisal angle very slightly rounded.

The crown tapers evenly to the narrow arc which describes the cementoenamel junction.

This design places the contact with adjoining teeth very near the incisal edge. The mandibular lateral incisor is similar. This arrangement is a radical departure from the form of the other teeth in the arch. When the incisal edges are worn by use, the incisal edge and contact areas become almost

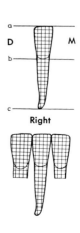

Right

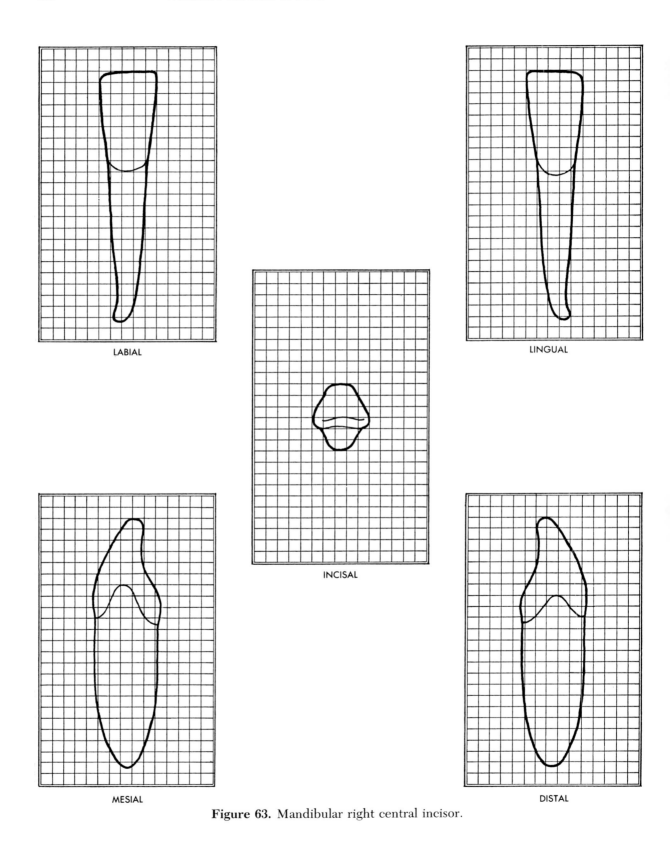

LABIAL

LINGUAL

INCISAL

MESIAL

DISTAL

Figure 63. Mandibular right central incisor.

continuous, with little or no escapement due to obliteration of embrasure space incisally.

The root outlines on the mesial and distal surfaces are continuous with the mesial and distal outlines of the crown. The apical third of the root comes to a rather fine taper, curving distally at the apical end. As heretofore mentioned, any root ending in a small taper may curve either mesially or distally. So many roots curve distally, however, that this curvature may be accepted as the general rule.

Lingual Aspect

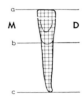

The drawing of this aspect is a reverse drawing of that of the labial aspect. There is one change: the cementoenamel junction is placed 0.5 mm. apically, making the crown 0.5 mm. longer on the lingual side.

Mesial Aspect

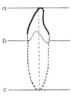

The mesial aspect demonstrates the tooth's greatest bulk.

The curvature labially and lingually of the cervical third of the crown above the cementoenamel junction is less than that found on the maxillary teeth.

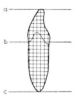

The outline of the labial face of the crown is straight, sloping rapidly from the greatest crest of curvature to the incisal edge. The lingual outline of the crown is concave above the smooth cingulum, a fact which makes the crown very slender at the middle third and incisal third. The incisal edge is rounded and lingual to the root axis. This last point should be noted as differing from maxillary anteriors except in the case of "hawkbills."

The curvature of the cementoenamel junction mesially is marked, curving incisally approximately one-third the length of the crown.

The root outlines on the mesial aspect drop straight down from the cervical line, keeping the root diameter labiolingually almost uniform in the cervical and middle thirds. The apical third tapers rapidly to a rounded end.

Distal Aspect

The outline of this aspect is a reverse drawing of that of the mesial aspect. The line describing the cervical curvature of the cementoenamel junction extends about 1 mm. less cervicoincisally.

Incisal Aspect

This aspect shows that the mandibular central incisor has almost bilateral symmetry. The mesial half of the crown is very much like the distal half.

The incisal edge is approximately at right angles to a line bisecting the crown labiolingually.

Note the comparison between the diameter of the crown labiolingually and its diameter mesiodistally.

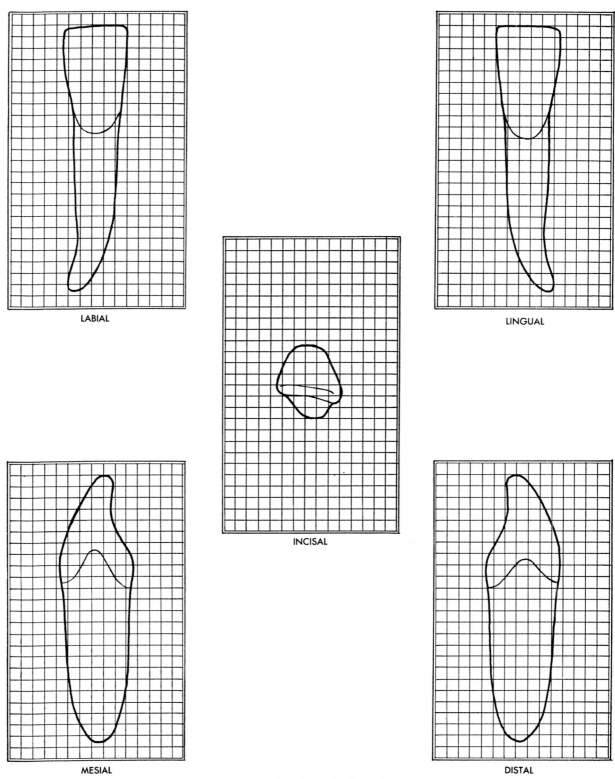

Figure 64. Mandibular right lateral incisor.

MANDIBULAR LATERAL INCISOR

The mandibular lateral or second incisor is the second mandibular tooth from the median line.

As this tooth supplements the central incisor in function, the functional form is similar.

Compare the graphs of the lateral incisor with those of the central incisor, observing the following variations:

The mandibular lateral incisor is slightly larger than the mandibular central (compare the measurements) but, in general, the outline form has a marked resemblance. The mandibular lateral incisor does not show the variations when compared to its neighboring central incisor that were observed when comparing the maxillary lateral incisor to the maxillary central. The size relationship is directly opposite, since the mandibular lateral incisor is always slightly larger than its neighboring central.

The labial and lingual outlines show the added 0.5 mm. of crown width mesiodistally to be added to the distal side. The crest of curvature distally, which of course represents the contact area, is a full millimeter distal to the cervical line, whereas the mesial crest is about 0.5 mm. mesial to the cervical line. The distal contact area is more cervical in location than the mesial contact area.

Except for dimensions there is no difference between the outlines mesially and distally of the central and lateral incisors. Even the cementoenamel curvature mesially and distally is similar in extent.

The incisal aspect provides the most certain test in the identification of this tooth. The incisal edge does not approach a ninety degree angle to a line bisecting the crown and root labiolingually as was found in the central incisor. The incisal edge has a more extreme angle and follows the curve of the mandibular arch, although the root axes labiolingually of the mandibular lateral and central incisors remain almost parallel in the alveolar process.

The root form is similar to the mandibular central incisor except for its greater length in most cases.

MANDIBULAR CANINE

The mandibular canine is the third mandibular tooth from the median line. It has the same function to perform as the maxillary canine, therefore its outlines from all aspects bear considerable resemblance.

Generally speaking, the mandibular canine crown is smoother in appearance than the maxillary canine crown, and looks slender in comparison.

The mandibular canine crown is narrower mesiodistally than that of the maxillary canine, although it is just as long in most instances and quite often is slightly longer. The labiolingual diameter of the crown is usually a fraction of a millimeter less. (Refer to page 26.)

The lingual surface of the crown is smoother in the mandibular canine with less cingulum development and less bulk to the marginal ridges than the maxillary canine. There is less curvature labially above the cervical line and also lingually, including the cingulum. This design is characteristic of all mandibular incisors. In fact, the lingual portion of the mandibular canine and the outline form of the tooth when viewed from the mesial aspect

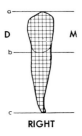

RIGHT

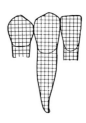

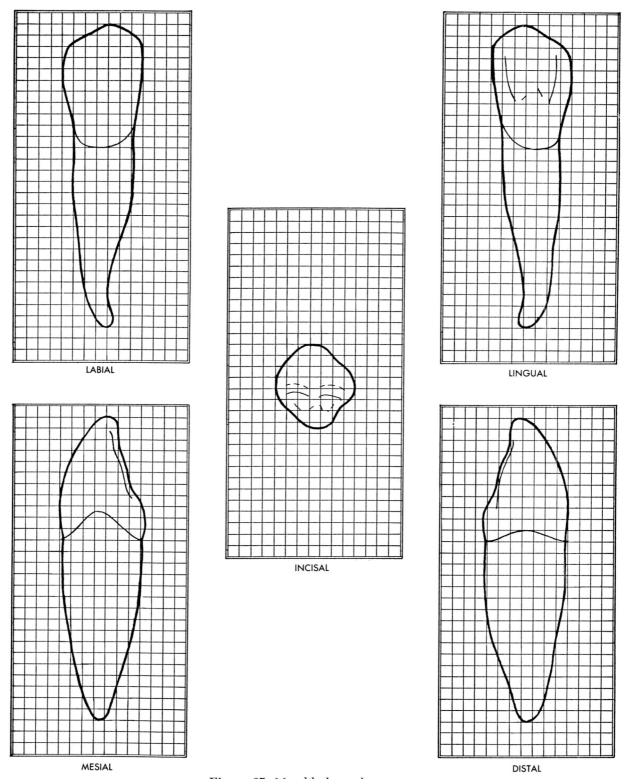

LABIAL

LINGUAL

INCISAL

MESIAL

DISTAL

Figure 65. Mandibular right canine.

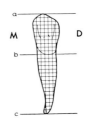

resemble the mandibular lateral incisor considerably. Compare Figure 64 with Figure 65.

The cusp of the mandibular canine is not so well developed as that of the maxillary canine, and the cusp ridges are thinner labiolingually.

The contact area levels are quite different mesially and distally, as was found in the maxillary canine, because they must contact a tooth of one kind mesially (lateral incisor) and one of another kind distally (first premolar). However, the mesial contact area of the mandibular canine is nearer the incisal angle than is the maxillary canine and the distal contact area is above the halfway mark from the cervical line labially to the cusp tip level.

In the reference drawing of the mandibular canine the root tip was made to curve mesially just to emphasize the possibility of variation in this respect.

When newly erupted, before the cusp has shown any wear, the crown of this tooth is often the longest in the mouth.

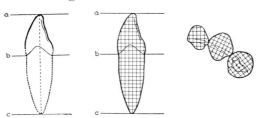

MANDIBULAR FIRST PREMOLAR

The mandibular first premolar is the fourth mandibular tooth from the median line and the first posterior tooth.

This tooth supplements both the canine and second premolar in function and, therefore, has some of the characteristics of each of them.

Although the first mandibular premolar has two cusps and corresponds to the second premolar more closely in size, its only functioning cusp, the buccal, is long, sharp and developed to resemble closely the cusp form of the canine. In addition, the outline form of the occlusal aspect is similar to that of the incisal aspect of a canine.

The single root is rounded, sometimes rather short, with an even taper.

Buccal Aspect

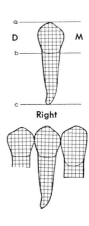

Right

The form of this tooth from the buccal aspect is nearly symmetrical bilaterally. The buccal cusp is large, pointed and well developed. The contact areas are broad, with the crests of curvature almost at the same level mesially and distally and at little more than half the distance from cervix to cusp tip. The outlines of mesial and distal surfaces from cervix to crests of curvature are slightly concave. The measurement of the crown mesiodistally at the cervical line is narrow when it is compared with the calibration at the contact areas.

The root presents an even taper from the crown to the apical third of the root. At that point it is much slenderer, curving distally at the apical end.

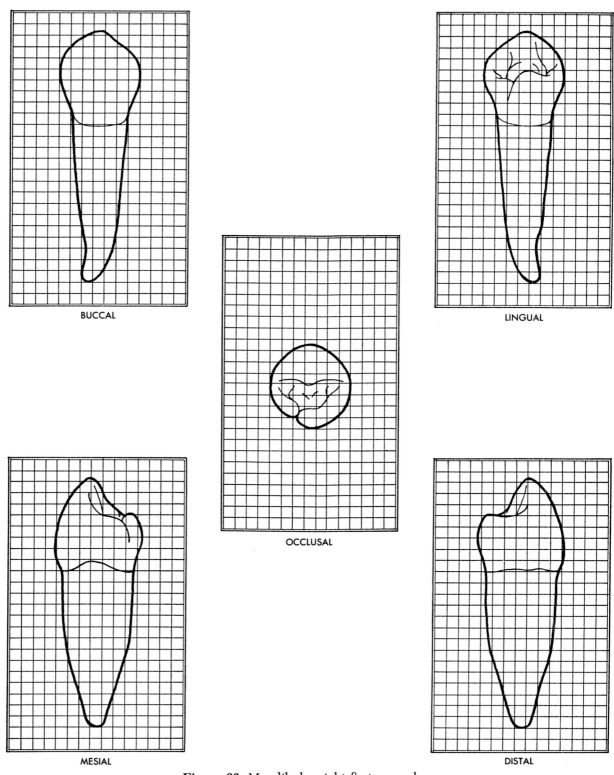

BUCCAL

LINGUAL

OCCLUSAL

MESIAL

DISTAL

Figure 66. Mandibular right first premolar.

Lingual Aspect

The outline of the tooth from the lingual aspect is a reverse outline to that viewed from the buccal. From this aspect the small, poorly developed lingual cusp is seen. The length and development of the lingual cusp will vary in different individuals. On the average, the lingual cusp will be a little more than half the height of the buccal cusp.

A feature of this tooth is the developmental groove to the mesial of the lingual cusp.

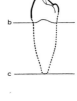

Mesial Aspect

Here we see a variation of functional design from that of maxillary posterior teeth, a variation which is characteristic of all mandibular posteriors; that is, a line bisecting the buccal cusp will more nearly approach the center axis of the root. The convexity of the lingual outline of the lingual cusp will be lingual to the lingual outline of the root.

The developmental groove mesially is in full view.

The line describing the cementoenamel junction mesially curves occlusally approximately 1 mm. only.

The lines describing the roots are almost straight from the cervix to a point half the root length, then taper markedly from that point to the apex.

It might be well at this point to repeat the important observations stated above.

When viewing mandibular posterior teeth from the mesial aspect, buccal cusps will more nearly approach the center of the root base than those of maxillary posterior teeth. Some mandibular first premolars may have the buccal cusp actually centered and in line with the root axis. The convexity of the lingual outline of lingual cusps of mandibular posterior teeth will be lingual to the lingual outlines of roots.

The crowns of maxillary posterior teeth, on the other hand, will show their cusps to be well within the outlines of the root "base" when the tooth is held with its axis in a vertical direction.

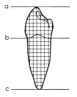

Distal Aspect

The outline of the distal aspect of this tooth is the reverse of that of the mesial aspect. There is no developmental groove, the marginal ridge is somewhat higher, and the cervical curvature is practically nil.

Occlusal Aspect

This aspect is almost circular in outline with an offset at the developmental groove mesially.

The distal outline is almost a semicircle from the crest of curvature buccally to the crest of curvature lingually. The mesial outline describes a smaller semicircular arc from the developmental groove mesially to the crest of curve buccally. This arrangement affords a smaller, more constricted contact area mesially, where this tooth contacts the canine, than the broad contact area distally where it contacts the second premolar.

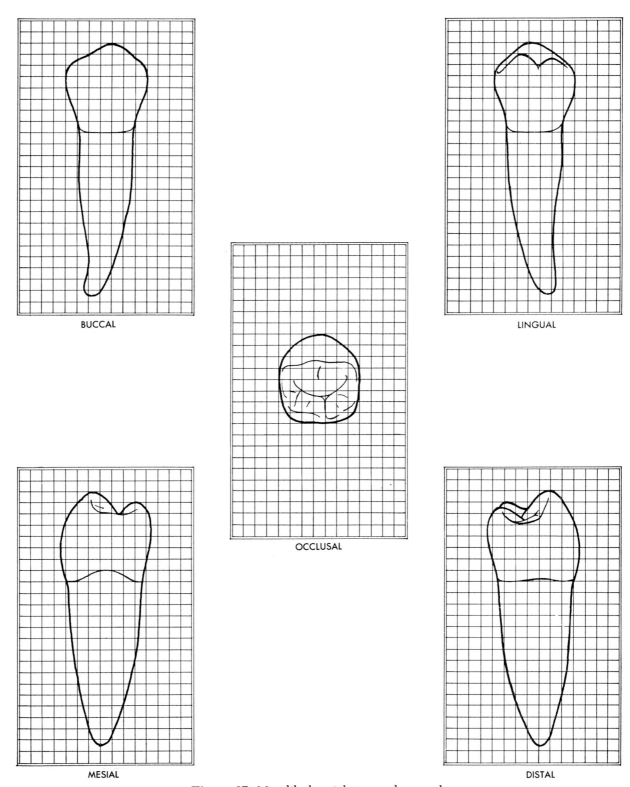

BUCCAL

LINGUAL

OCCLUSAL

MESIAL

DISTAL

Figure 67. Mandibular right second premolar.

MANDIBULAR SECOND PREMOLAR

The mandibular second premolar is the fifth mandibular tooth from the median line. Although the mesiodistal measurements of crown and root are about the same as the first mandibular premolar, it is larger and has better development in other respects.

There are two common forms which this tooth assumes. The first, which is illustrated here and which occurs most often, is the three-cusp type. The second is the two-cusp type which has a single lingual cusp. The two types differ only in occlusal design. The outlines in other respects are similar.

The root of the mandibular second premolar is larger and longer than the first premolar. A study of radiograms of the teeth in dental examinations will show the root longer than those of mandibular first molars in many instances. In describing the separate aspects of this tooth, direct comparison with the first premolar will be made.

Buccal Aspect

The buccal cusp is shorter than the first premolar and not so pointed. The root is longer. The outline otherwise is similar.

Lingual Aspect

The outline of this aspect is just the reverse of the buccal aspect. The two lingual cusps may be seen below the level of the buccal cusp.

The mesiolingual cusp is somewhat larger than the distolingual cusp.

Mesial Aspect

The comparison here shows the same relationship of crown to root and the same general outline as the first premolar except there is no developmental groove mesiolingually, the marginal ridge is higher, and the lingual cusp shown is much nearer the length of the buccal cusp.

Distal Aspect

From this aspect all three of the cusps may be seen. In other respects, the drawing is a reverse picture of the mesial aspect.

Occlusal Aspect

The occlusal aspect is quite different from that of the first mandibular premolar. The only similarity is the outline of the buccal third. The contact areas are broad and flat and the outline of the three cusps, which is lingual to the buccal third of the crown, is quite square. The central pit, where the developmental occlusal grooves join, is off-center distally.

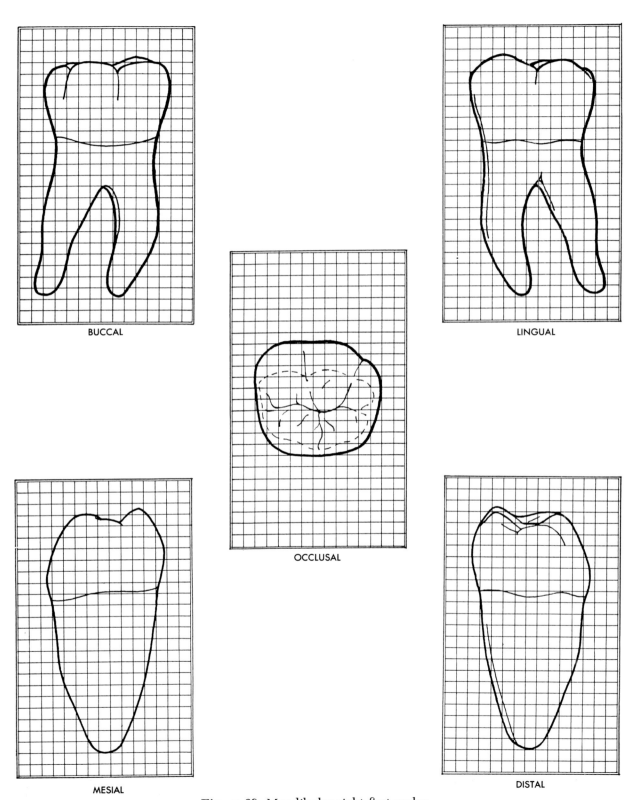

BUCCAL

LINGUAL

OCCLUSAL

MESIAL

DISTAL

Figure 68. Mandibular right first molar.

MANDIBULAR FIRST MOLAR

The mandibular first molar is the sixth mandibular tooth from the median line. Normally it is the largest tooth in the mandibular arch. It has five well-developed cusps: two buccal and two lingual cusps and a distal cusp.

There are two well-developed roots, one mesial and one distal, which are very broad buccolingually and well separated at the apices (Figs. 68, 69, 70, and 71).

Buccal Aspect

The line describing the cementoenamel junction on the buccal surface is a gently curving line dipping root-wise. The point of greatest curvature is centered buccally.

The *mesial outline* of the *crown* is nearly straight from the cervix to the contact area, which is approximately at the junction of the occlusal and the middle third of the crown. The convexity of the contact area joins the rounded outline of the mesiobuccal cusp.

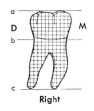

Right

The *distal outline* of the *crown* is similar to the mesial outline. The crest of curvature at the contact area is a little lower because of the fact that the distal cusp, whose convex outline it joins, is shorter than the mesiobuccal cusp.

The two *buccal cusps* and the *distal cusp* may be completely outlined from this aspect. The two buccal cusps are separated by the mesiobuccal developmental groove; the distobuccal cusp and the distal cusp are separated by the distobuccal groove.

The two buccal cusps are almost the same width mesiodistally, making up together almost 80 per cent of the total mesiodistal width of the buccal surface of the crown. The distal cusp is much smaller, making up the remainder or about 20 per cent.

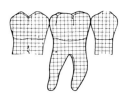

Since the lingual cusps are longer they can be seen from the buccal aspect when the tooth is posed vertically.

Although the outlines of all the cusps are convex, the buccal cusps of the mandibular first molar are not pointed. They appear flat in comparison with the lingual cusps.

Both *roots* are in view from this aspect.

The mesial outline of the mesial root is concave below the cemento-enamel junction to a point about halfway down the root. This point is on a line with the junction of crown and root mesially. Then the line becomes convex, straightening as it approaches the apex of the mesial root. The apex of this root is almost on a line with the mesiobuccal groove of the crown.

The distal outline of the distal root is also concave below the crown cervix, but changes to a convex line before reaching the middle portion of the root. It changes again to a concave line before it completes the rounded apex of the distal root. The center of the apex of the distal root is on a line with the crest of curvature distal to the distal cusp of the crown.

The drawing of the roots is completed by outlining the distal of the mesial root and the mesial of the distal root, joining the outlines at the point

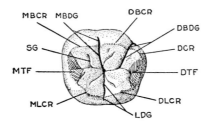

Figure 69. Mandibular first molar—occlusal aspect. *DBCR*, Distobuccal cusp ridge; *DBDG*, distobuccal developmental groove; *DCR*, distal cusp ridge; *DTF*, distal triangular fossa (shaded area); *DLCR*, distolingual cusp ridge; *LDG*, lingual developmental groove; *MLCR*, mesiolingual cusp ridge; *MTF*, mesial triangular fossa (shaded area); *SG*, a supplemental groove; *MBCR*, mesiobuccal cusp ridge; *MBDG*, mesiobuccal developmental groove.

Figure 70. Mandibular first molar—occlusal aspect. Shaded area—central fossa; *CP*, central pit; *DMR*, distal marginal ridge; *DP*, distal pit; *CDG*, central developmental groove; *MP*, mesial pit; *MMR*, mesial marginal ridge.

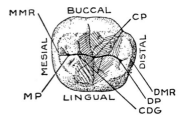

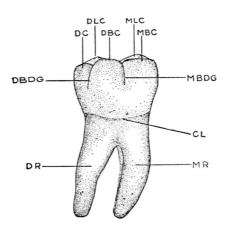

Figure 71. Mandibular first molar—buccal aspect. *MBDG*, Mesiobuccal developmental groove; *CL*, cervical line; *MR*, mesial root; *DR*, distal root; *DBDG*, distobuccal developmental groove; *DC*, distal cusp; *DLC*, distolingual cusp; *DBC*, distobuccal cusp; *MLC*, mesiolingual cusp; *MBC*, mesiobuccal cusp.

of bifurcation, 3 or 4 mm. below the cementoenamel junction of the crown centrally and buccally. Each root will be approximately 4 mm. thick at the bifurcation and 2 mm. thick near the apex.

A line bisecting the mesial root will be curved, and one bisecting the distal root will be almost straight.

Lingual Aspect

The outline of the lingual aspect is a reverse outline to that of the buccal aspect except for the following details:

The line describing the cementoenamel junction is an uneven, waving line.

The two lingual cusps make up most of the occlusal outline, showing the mesiolingual cusp to be the wider of the two.

Part of the distal cusp is visible and also part of the two buccal cusps just beyond the sulcus between the two lingual cusps. A short developmental groove is shown separating the lingual cusps. Sometimes there is only a dip in the enamel with no developmental groove in evidence.

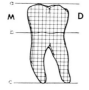

Mesial Aspect

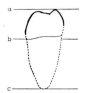

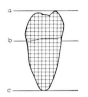

The cervical line mesially is only slightly curved, ending about 1 mm. higher lingually than buccally.

The *buccal outline* of the *crown* is quite convex above the cemento-enamel junction to a point about half the crown length. The line becomes straighter from this point to the buccal cusp. It will be noted that the curvature outward buccally just above the root is about 0.5 mm.

The *lingual outline* of the *crown* is convex in its entirety, with the crest of curvature at about the center of the middle third of the crown. (This should be compared with the buccal outline where the crest of curvature is at the junction of cervical and middle thirds.)

The crown drawing of the mesial aspect is completed by the outlines of the buccal cusp and the lingual cusp with the mesial marginal ridge. The buccal cusp is rather flat, and the lingual cusp is sharp, with greater cusp height.

The outline of the mesial root only is visible from the mesial aspect because it is broader than the distal root.

The *buccal outline* of the *root* drops down almost straight from the cementoenamel junction to a point about half the root length. Then it curves sharply, continuing as a line almost straight from that point to the bluntly rounded apex directly centered below the crown.

The *lingual outline* of the *root* starts at the cementoenamel junction as a direct continuation of the lingual outline of the crown with no offset as found on the buccal. The curvature of the lingual outline of the root is very gradual as it comes down to join the rounded apex.

Distal Aspect

The outline of the distal aspect is a reverse outline of that of the mesial aspect except for the following details:

Most of the occlusal surface is visible from this aspect. Therefore, an outline of all the cusps is shown. The distal cusp is slightly off-center to the buccal.

The cervical line is uneven, dipping rootwise below the center of the crown buccolingually.

Since the distal root is narrower buccolingually than the mesial root, a line is drawn parallel and just inside the lingual outline of the mesial root to show this difference in width.

Occlusal Aspect

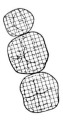

The points to be brought out on the drawing of this aspect are the relative positions of the contact areas, the relative positions of the cusps to each other, the design and direction of the grooves on the occlusal surface, and the diameter of the crown mesiodistally as compared to the diameter buccolingually. (See page 72 and Fig. 128.)

The following points are to be noted especially:

The occlusal surface between the cusp ridges, with its sulci and grooves, is placed lingual to the center of the crown. In other words, more of the buccal surface of the crown shows from this aspect than the lingual surface. (*Maxillary* molars have their occlusal surfaces more directly centered over the root base.)

There are two large buccal cusps and one distal cusp (not three evenly divided buccal cusps).

The distal contact area is located on the distal cusp.

The crown tapers lingually from the contact areas.

There are two lingual cusps, making five cusps altogether.

MANDIBULAR SECOND MOLAR

The mandibular second molar is the seventh mandibular tooth from the median line.

Because it supplements the first mandibular molar in function, its design is similar. Compare the graph drawings of the mandibular second molar with those of the first molar, observing the following variations:

Buccal Aspect

The crown is not so long cervico-occlusally.

The two buccal cusps are almost equal in size.

The two roots are not formed so heavily; the roots are more nearly parallel to each other and have less spread.

The distal root is longer than the mesial root.

Lingual Aspect

The drawing of this aspect is a reverse outline to that of the buccal aspect. Since the tips of the lingual cusp are higher than the buccal cusps, only the lingual cusps are in view. They are almost equal in size. The mesiolingual cusp is usually a trifle wider mesiodistally.

Because of the twist of the mesial root, part of the distal portion may be seen through the bifurcation of the mesial and distal roots.

Mesial Aspect

The mesial aspect of the mandibular second molar varies little from that of the first molar, except for the difference in the root lengths and the height of crown portions.

The distal root is longer than the mesial root on the second molar, whereas the opposite situation is true of the first molar.

Distal Aspect

Here also we find little variation from the outline of the mandibular first molar. There is no distal cusp, and the outline of the cementoenamel junction is less distinct.

It is interesting to note that part of the mesial root may be seen from this aspect on the buccal side; on the first molar the opposite is true—it is to be seen on the lingual side. This proves the observation that the crowns of these teeth are set at different angulations to the roots.

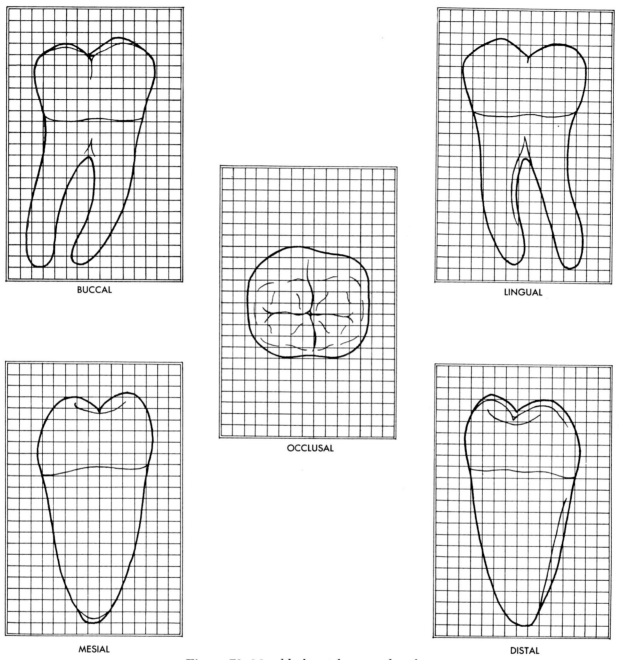

BUCCAL

LINGUAL

OCCLUSAL

MESIAL

DISTAL

Figure 72. Mandibular right second molar.

Occlusal Aspect

From this point of view, considerable difference may be seen between the two designs of mandibular molars.

Instead of the five cusps of varying sizes in the first molar, we have four cusps nearly equal in size. This centers the occlusal grooves between the cusps, a condition causing them to meet evenly at the central pit which is centered in the occlusal surface of the crown of the second molar.

An outline of the occlusal surface at the points of cusps and marginal ridges will almost portray a rectangle.

The buccal outline of this aspect differs somewhat from that of the first molar. There is one developmental groove centered buccally which divides the two buccal cusps rather evenly although the mesiobuccal cusp is somewhat larger.

From the occlusal aspect, the buccal and lingual outlines of the crown show a tapered effect from the mesial portion back toward the distal portion. All mandibular molars have this characteristic.

MANDIBULAR THIRD MOLAR

The mandibular third molar is the eighth and last mandibular tooth from the median line.

Because it supplements the second molar in function, the fundamental design is similar. The tooth is smaller and not so well developed.

The mandibular third molar varies considerably in different individuals, presenting many anomalies both in form and position, tending to be oversized and malaligned. The illustrations will demonstrate an average mandibular third molar which would occlude properly with its antagonist in the maxillary arch as pictured in this atlas.

In making comparisons with the second molar, the following points are to be observed.

Buccal Aspect

The crown is about the same length cervico-occlusally but is narrower mesiodistally.

The roots are fused together, functioning as one large root, and they are shorter cervicoapically.

The fused roots divide sufficiently at the apex to form two distinct apices.

The outline mesially and distally of the fused roots has a more extreme slant toward the distal, placing the apices of the roots in a more distal relationship to the center of the crown.

Lingual Aspect

There is no outstanding variation here except those mentioned under buccal aspect.

Mesial Aspect

The distal root apex cannot be seen. Except for this detail, the only variations in the design of this tooth from that of the second molar are differences in measurement.

Distal Aspect

The outline of the distal aspect is quite similar to that of the second molar, making allowances for a narrower crown buccolingually and shorter roots.

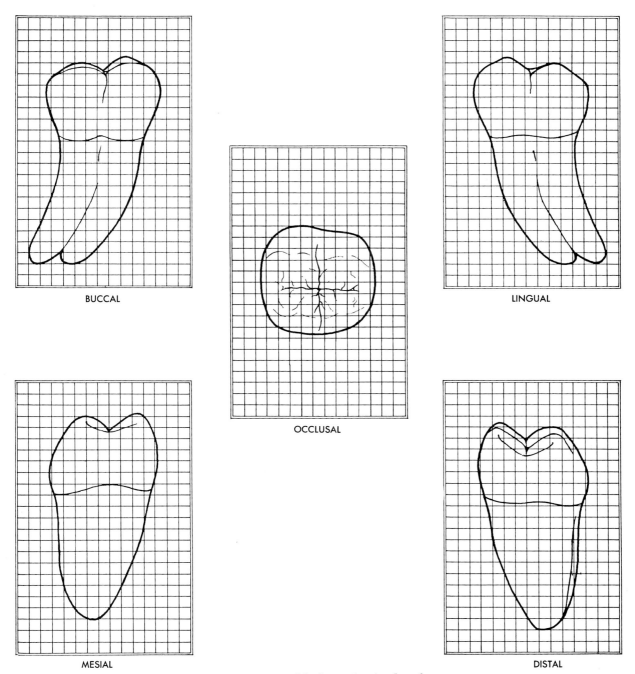

Figure 73. Mandibular right third molar.

BUCCAL

OCCLUSAL

LINGUAL

MESIAL

DISTAL

Occlusal Aspect

A drawing of this view is very similar to that of the second molar.

The crown is shorter mesiodistally and narrower buccolingually.

The crown tapers more distally, and the "line angles" are more rounded. This places the distobuccal cusp and the distolingual cusp close together.

A greater number of supplemental grooves will be in evidence occlusally.

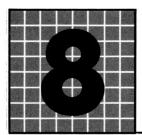

Plaster Sculpture

LABORATORY TECHNIQUE DESCRIBED AND ILLUSTRATED

It is taken for granted that the reader is now familiar with two dimensional tooth form (drawing). In order to achieve proper perspective, it is necessary to progress to the production of three dimensional form.

The logical material for our purpose is plaster of Paris. The material permits the drawing of tooth form on its surface, establishing measurements and proportion; when the carving progresses, the material will serve as a record of progress. Smaller block material, like the Ivorine sticks for carving teeth natural size (see page 102), is too small for instruction and carving practice for beginners. The plaster block will allow the drawing of tooth design on its sides, and the material, during the carving and finishing process, makes a permanent record, easily seen, of the student's work.

The plaster block should be just large enough to accommodate the drawings previously studied, namely, the scale of ⅛ inch to equal 1 mm. The carvings when finished will be approximately three diameters when compared with the measurements of natural teeth.

Plaster blocks are required measuring 4 × 1¾ inches (Figs. 76 *a* and 78).

Figures 78 to 85 demonstrate the steps in carving plaster models of teeth from the plaster blocks.

In this course of plaster sculpture, the crowns of the teeth and at least the cervical third of the roots are to be carved out, leaving the remainder of the block as a heavy base for the carving. The illustrations of plaster carvings on the following pages, made according to the technique advocated in this book, include one-half the root length. It is impossible to reproduce the form of the cervical third of the crown without including a goodly portion of the root in the finished carving.

Anterior Tooth

Mark the four longest sides of a plaster block—labial, lingual, mesial and distal. Use a 6-inch rule and measure off ¼ inch all around the top of

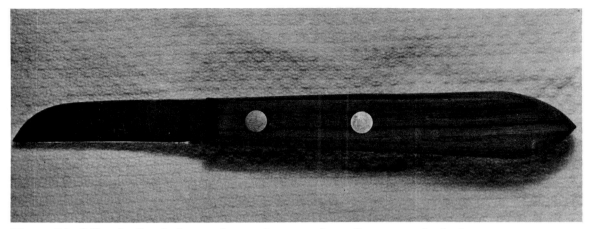

Figure 74. Office knife which may be used to complete all carvings, both three diameter and normal size. (S.S.W. Dental Mfg. Co.)

the plaster block. Drawings and cutouts will be made below this line, which allows a margin of safety. Use a sharp-pointed pencil for marking. If the incisal and occlusal outlines are placed at the same level on each block, the length of all carvings will be uniform.

Draw the labial aspect of the tooth on the labial face of the block, starting the incisal surface at the ¼-inch margin and completing the drawing of the labial aspect of the crown and root. Draw a line around the block above the apex of the root wherever it is desired to terminate the root carving. The remainder of the surface of the block between this line and the lower border will outline the base which is left intact (Fig. 76 *a*). Usually one-half the root length is carved out on the plaster carvings (somewhat less than illustration; see plaster carvings).

The lingual or opposite surface of the crown and root is outlined in the same manner on the opposite face of the block.

A plaster saw blade is now used in the mechanical saw frame to cut the plaster away from the outside of the outline of the crown and root form; it is best to saw a little away from the tooth outline (Fig. 78).

The office knife is used next to complete the cut, the student carving to the outline of the labial and lingual aspects accurately *without allowing any plaster outside of the outline at any point from the labial surface clear through to the lingual* (Fig. 76 *b;* also Fig. 80).

The office knife is used as a scraper or plane to get the sides smooth and accurate as to scale. Unless these cuts are made accurately and smoothly, the measurements will be lost when the blocking-in process is completed. A caliper is used to calibrate the work and to maintain accuracy. The finished operation should have the appearance of a planed surface.

After the first operation is completed, draw the mesial and distal view of the crown and root on the cut sides (Fig. 76 *c*).

Continue as before with the saw and knife until the crown and root are blocked out on a plaster base as in Figure 76 *d*.

If the second operation has been done properly, the measurements of the block tooth will be correct to scale.

The labial or buccal, lingual, mesial and distal outlines are now accurately portrayed. When this blocked-out carving is viewed from the incisal or occlusal, however, it is seen to be angular. The incisal or occlusal aspect, as outlined in the illustrations of tooth form, is most valuable from this point.

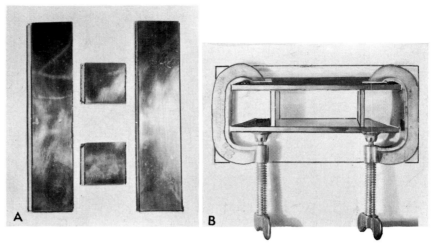

Figure 75. A brass mold quickly assembled, easily cleaned and almost indestructible is pictured above. The plaster blocks will measure exactly 4 × 1¾ × 1¾ inches and will come out clean and smooth.

A. The mold is made of pieces of standard brass "strip," 1¾ × ¼ inch; two pieces 8 inches long and two pieces square (1¾ × 1¾ inches).

B. The brass strips are placed edgewise on a piece of glass, making an enclosure by placing the square pieces at right angles to the longer pieces, and 4 inches apart. The boxing is held together by means of two 2½-inch iron clamps.

The mold parts should be thoroughly cleaned and wiped with a damp cloth after each pouring.

The "blocked-in" carving should have all measurements correct when checked with a caliper or Boley gauge. Angles are now removed and the carving completed by scraping and cutting until the proper tooth form is reproduced.

In a study of this kind, one cannot have too many visual aids. In this book, complete illustration was carefully planned, but other visual aids must be furnished by the instructor or the student himself. (See Fig. 89.) Carved models or tooth specimens should be available so that the student may observe perspective and the effect of three dimensional forms.

Plaster carvings of the eight typical forms which are finished according to recommended measurements may be obtained from the Columbia Dentoform Corporation if reference models are desired. Since they show the finished carvings in three dimensions they are quite useful when finishing blocked-in carvings.

In this work, as in any sculpture, a three dimensional model of some sort is necessary to acquire the proper perspective.

By observing an illustration of the incisal or occlusal aspect or by observing a completed carving, using it as a model, it is possible with practice to improve the anatomy, using the office knife as a carving instrument, until the piece has the characteristics and curves of a natural tooth (Fig. 76 e).

Posterior Tooth

The blocking-in process is done in the same manner when one is carving a posterior tooth with multicusps and multiroots except that allowance must be made for the flare of the roots; the student should be careful not to cut straight down from the crown cervix as is done with the single rooted tooth. Also, the occlusal surface is left flat on a level with the highest point of the cusps until the tooth is blocked in (Fig. 77). Then the cusp carving is completed while the other details of curvature are being finished.

This fact must always be kept in mind when carving teeth or parts of teeth: There are no actual points or angles on any human tooth in the true sense of the word. If a section were made of any part of a tooth, no matter how large or small, the piece cut off would be a section of a spheroid of large or small dimension.

In other words, an outline of any aspect of a tooth will describe arcs of circles, and no actual points or angles will be found. Therefore, in carving a tooth no sharp angles or points should remain on the finished piece. This suggestion should be heeded, particularly when one is carving occlusal surfaces of posterior teeth. Sulci, transverse ridges, etc., exhibit slopes which are convex, but beware of the so-called "planes of occlusion." *If flat planes occur on the occlusal surfaces of teeth, it is always the result of wear or accident.*

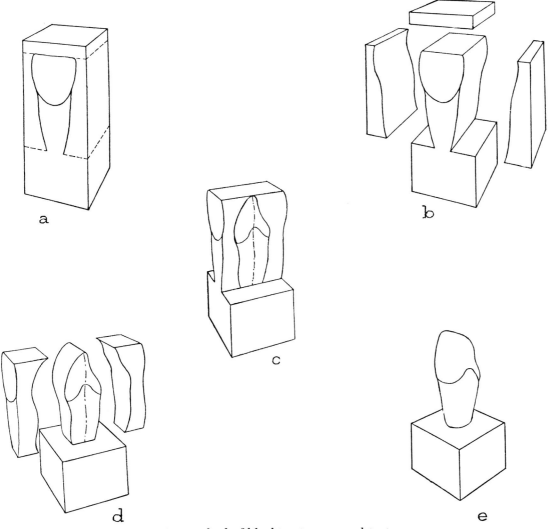

Figure 76. Method of blocking in a central incisor.

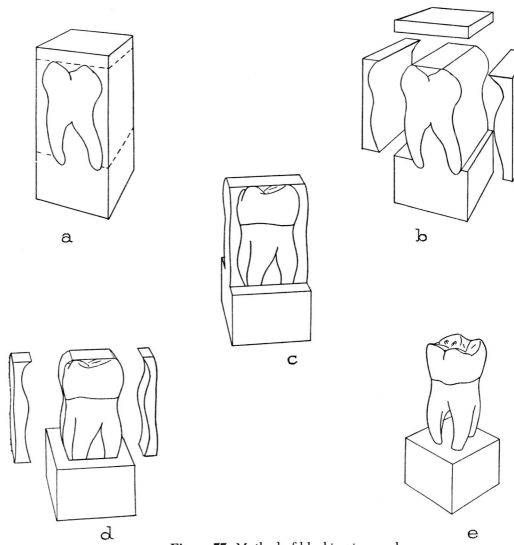

Figure 77. Method of blocking in a molar.

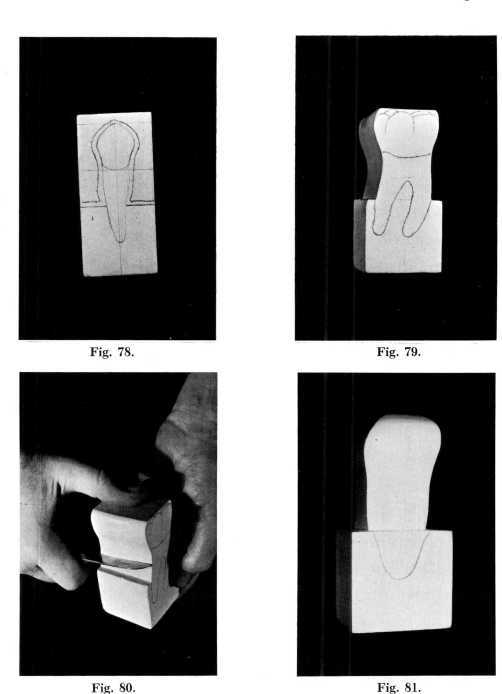

Fig. 78.   Fig. 79.

Fig. 80.   Fig. 81.

Figure 78. Plaster block with drawing for the first cut in blocking in the carving. Notice the irregular outline beyond the drawing which represents the saw cut removing excess plaster. Maxillary premolar.

Figure 79. The first cut completed on mandibular first molar.

Figure 80. Completing the first cut, using the knife as a plane. This operation is not complete until the caliper registers the exact measurement as represented by the drawing on both sides of the block.

Figure 81. Second cut completed. The carving is now "blocked in."

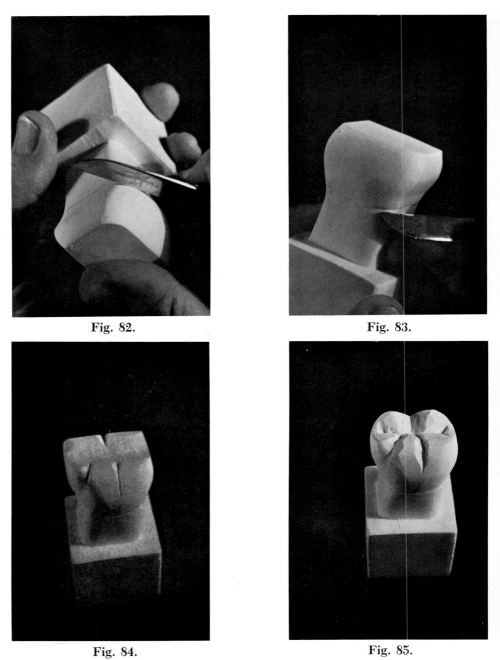

Fig. 82.

Fig. 83.

Fig. 84.

Fig. 85.

Figure 82. "Rounding the first corner," using the knife as a plane; rotating the block and scraping until the desired shape is produced.

Figure 83. *The cervical outline must be kept at all times.* First it is marked with pencil and then engraved with the knife. Whenever it seems necessary to erase it in changing the carving, it must be restored immediately at that location so that the complete cervical marking is never lost (Fig. 103).

Figure 84. The buccal portion of the crown has been shaped and notches cut to represent developmental grooves and cusp areas. Note how the occlusal portion has been scooped out roughly on a level with future marginal ridges.

Figure 85. The crown with its occlusal form is now "roughed in." Refer to page 97 for finished carving.

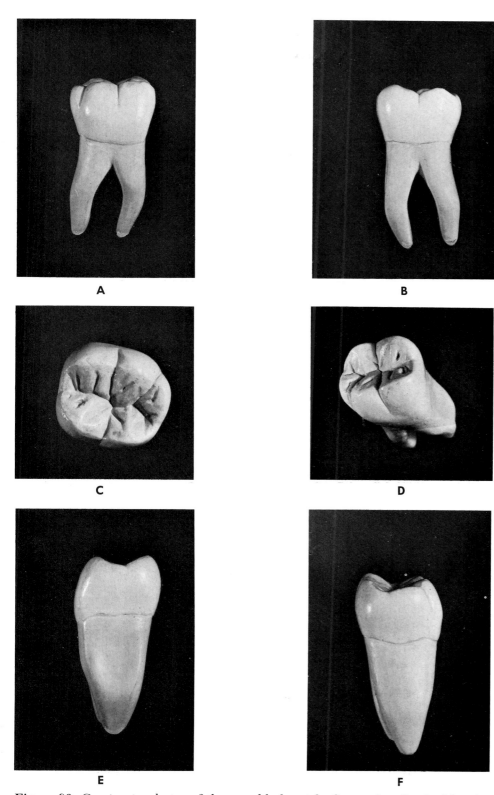

A

B

C

D

E

F

Figure 86. Carving in plaster of the mandibular right first molar, finished by the author to the scale of one-eighth inch equals one millimeter.

Figures 79 through 85 illustrate various steps in the carving procedure except for the finishing of roots as completed in this figure. *A,* Buccal aspect; *B,* lingual aspect; *C,* straight occlusal view; *D,* a perspective view from the occlusal aspect; *E,* mesial aspect; *F,* distal aspect.

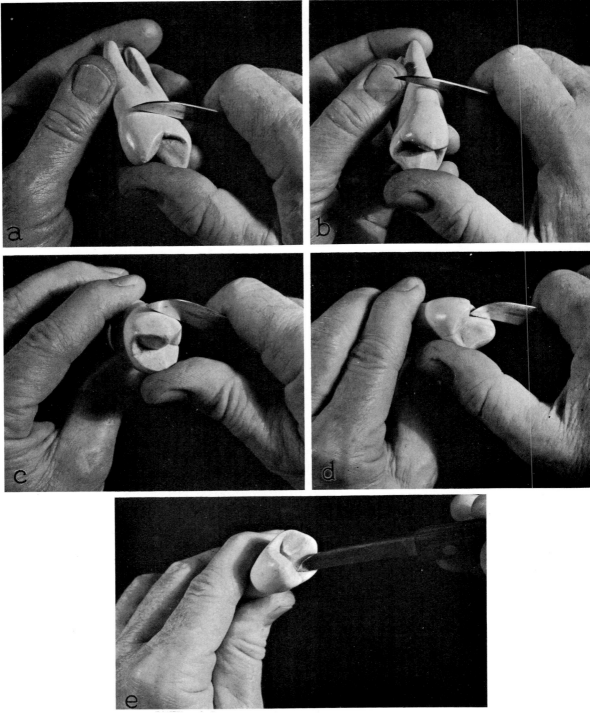

Figure 87. Demonstrating the use of the office knife as a carving instrument. Use the knife mostly as a plane, dragging the blade forward toward the operator. A variation in the pressure used will govern the speed of trimming. The point of the blade and the edge near the point is properly shaped for cutting action on the occlusal surfaces or wherever necessary.

MAXILLARY RIGHT CENTRAL INCISOR

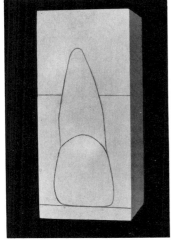

1. Drawing on block.

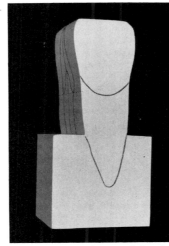

2. First cut from labial to lingual.

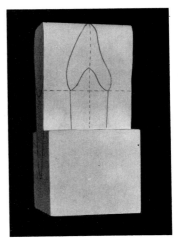

3. Drawing after first cut—Figure 76, c.

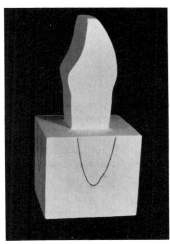

4. Mesial view after second cut.

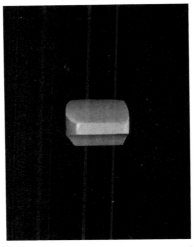

5. Incisal view after second cut.

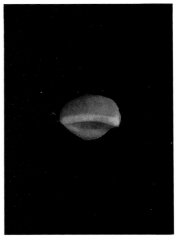

6. Incisal view of finished carving.

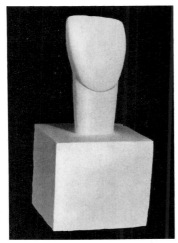

7. Labial view of finished carving.

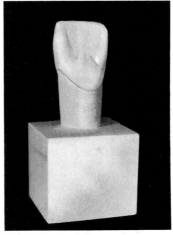

8. Lingual view of finished carving.

MAXILLARY RIGHT LATERAL INCISOR

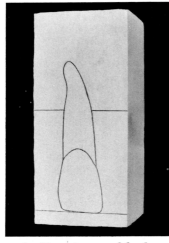

1. Drawing on block.

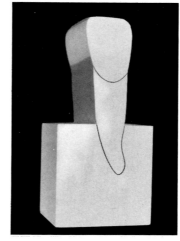

2. First cut from labial to lingual.

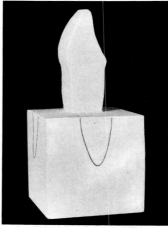

3. View after second cut.

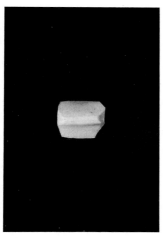

4. Incisal view after second cut.

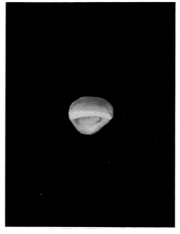

5. Incisal view of finished carving.

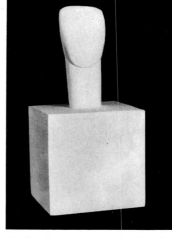

6. Labial view of finished carving.

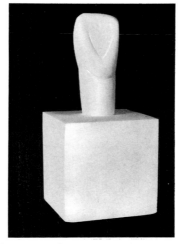

7. Lingual view of finished carving.

MAXILLARY RIGHT CANINE

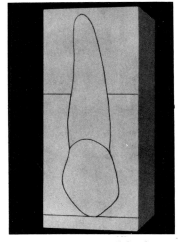

1. Drawing on block.

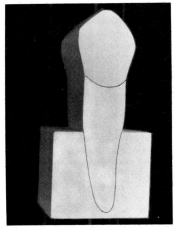

2. First cut from labial to lingual.

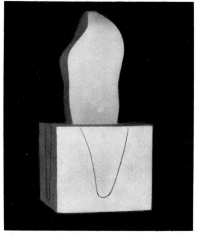

3. Second cut mesial to distal.

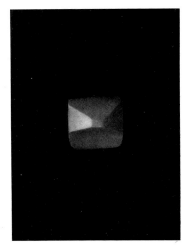

4. Incisal view after second cut.

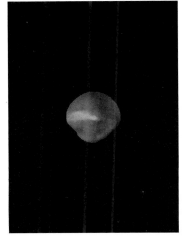

5. Incisal view of finished carving.

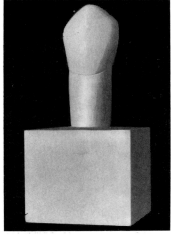

6. Labial view of finished carving.

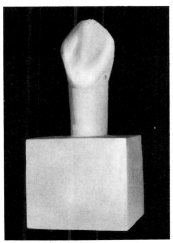

7. Lingual view of finished carving.

MAXILLARY RIGHT FIRST PREMOLAR

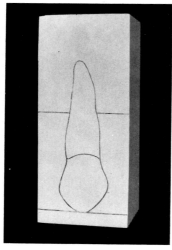

1. Drawing on block.

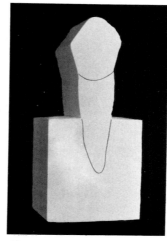

2. First cut from buccal to lingual.

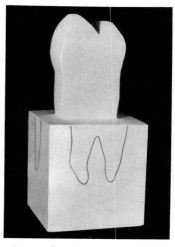

3. Second cut mesial to distal.

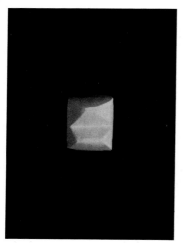

4. Occlusal view after second cut.

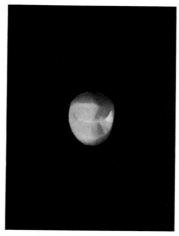

5. Occlusal view of finished carving.

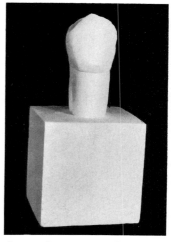

6. Buccal view of finished carving.

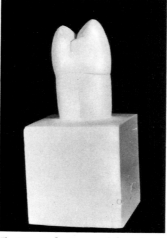

7. Mesial view of finished carving.

MAXILLARY RIGHT SECOND PREMOLAR

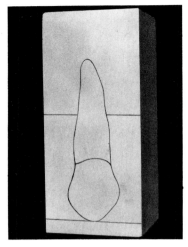

1. Drawing on block.

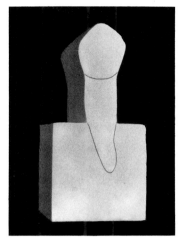

2. First cut from buccal to lingual.

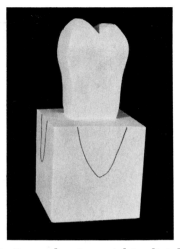

3. Second cut mesial to distal.

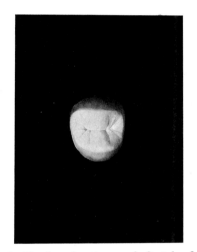

4. Occlusal view of finished carving.

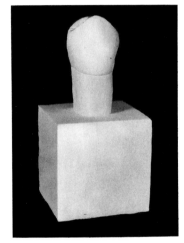

5. Buccal view of finished carving.

MAXILLARY RIGHT FIRST MOLAR

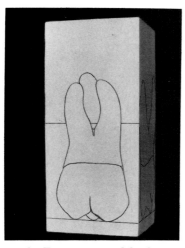

1. Drawing on block.

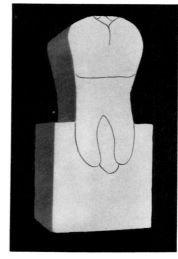

2. First cut from buccal to lingual.

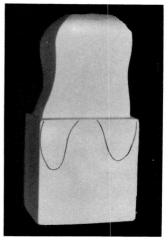

3. Second cut mesial to distal.

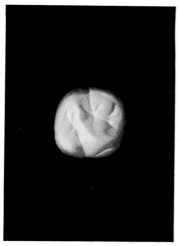

4. Occlusal view of finished carving.

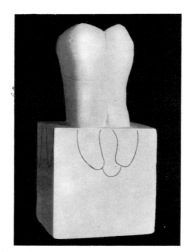

5. Buccal view of finished carving.

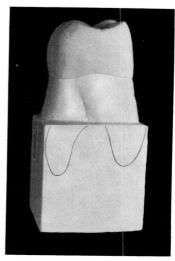

6. Mesial view of finished carving.

MAXILLARY RIGHT SECOND MOLAR

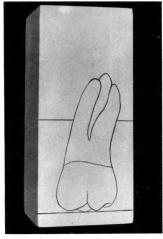

1. Drawing on block.

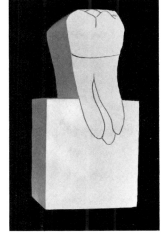

2. First cut buccal to lingual.

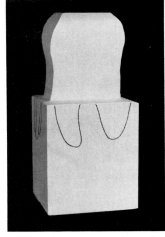

3. Second cut mesial to distal.

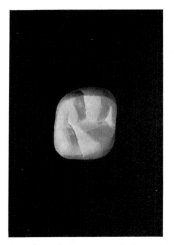

4. Occlusal view of finished carving.

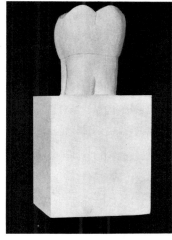

5. Buccal view of finished carving.

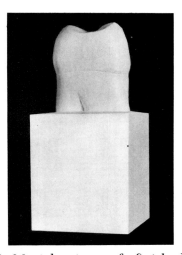

6. Mesial view of finished carving.

MANDIBULAR RIGHT CENTRAL INCISOR

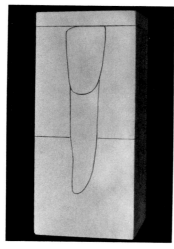

1. Drawing on block.

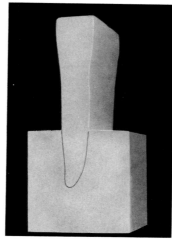

2. First cut from labial to lingual.

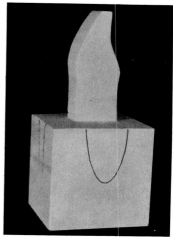

3. Second cut mesial to distal.

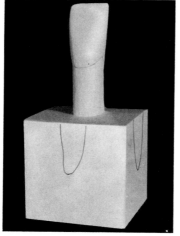

4. Labial view of finished carving.

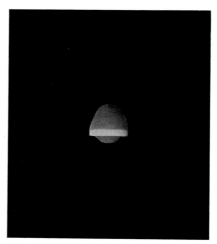

5. Incisal view of finished carving.

MANDIBULAR RIGHT LATERAL INCISOR

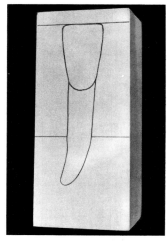

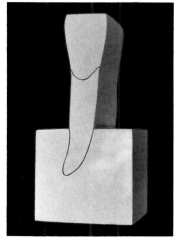

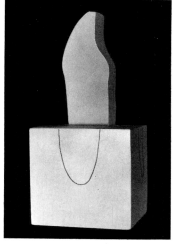

1. Drawing on block.

2. First cut labial to lingual.

3. Second cut mesial to distal.

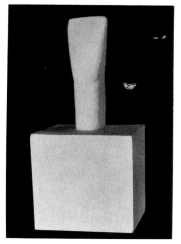

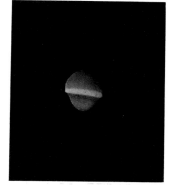

4. Labial view of finished
   carving.

5. Incisal view of finished
   carving.

MANDIBULAR RIGHT CANINE

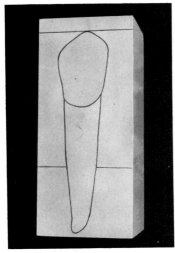

1. Drawing on block.

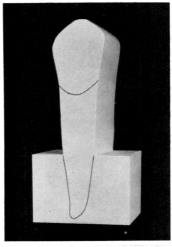

2. First cut from labial to lingual.

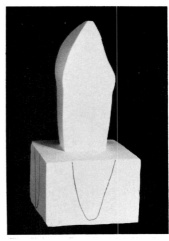

3. Second cut mesial to distal.

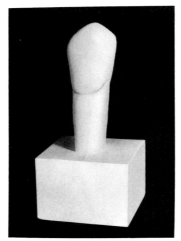

4. Labial view of finished carving.

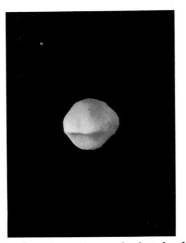

5. Incisal view of finished carving.

MANDIBULAR RIGHT FIRST PREMOLAR

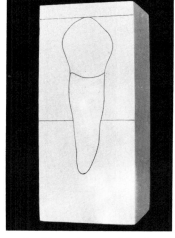

1. Drawing on block.

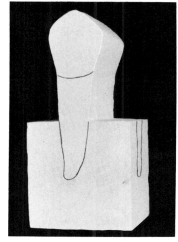

2. First cut from buccal to lingual.

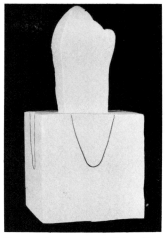

3. Second cut mesial to distal.

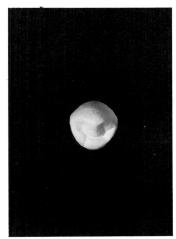

4. Occlusal view of finished carving.

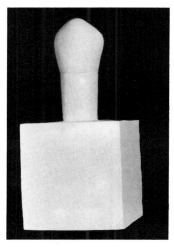

5. Buccal view of finished carving.

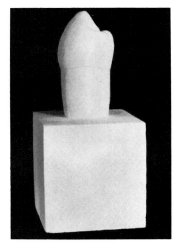

6. Mesial view of finished carving.

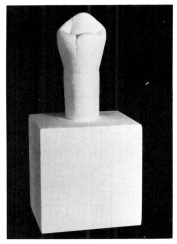

7. Lingual view of finished carving.

MANDIBULAR RIGHT SECOND PREMOLAR

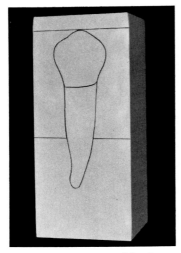

1. Drawing on block.

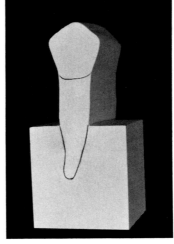

2. First cut buccal to lingual.

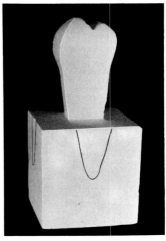

3. Second cut mesial to distal.

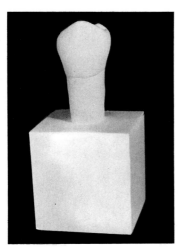

4. Buccal view of finished carving.

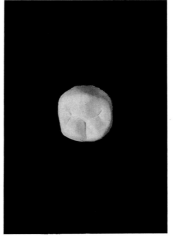

5. Occlusal view of finished carving.

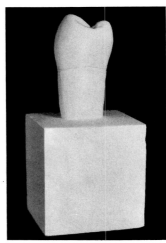

6. Mesial view of finished carving.

MANDIBULAR RIGHT FIRST MOLAR

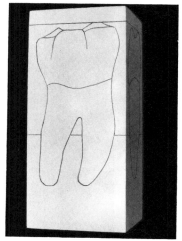

1. Drawing on block.

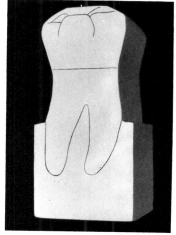

2. First cut from buccal to lingual.

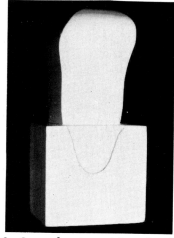

3. Second cut mesial to distal.

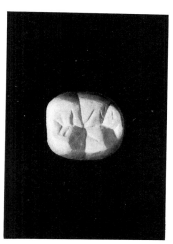

4. Occlusal view of finished carving.

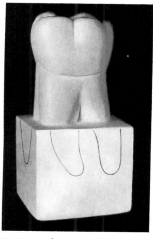

5. Buccal view of finished carving.

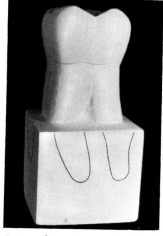

6. Lingual view of finished carving.

MANDIBULAR RIGHT SECOND MOLAR

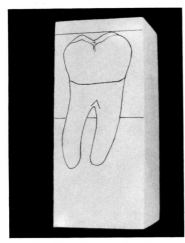

1. Drawing on block.

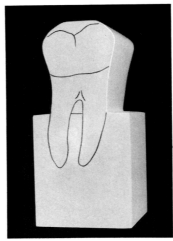

2. First cut buccal to lingual.

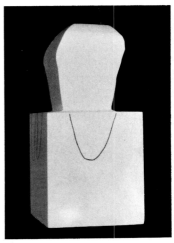

3. Second cut mesial to distal.

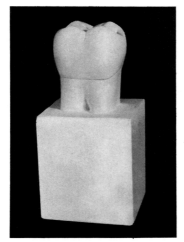

4. Buccal view of finished carving.

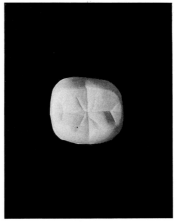

5. Occlusal view of finished carving.

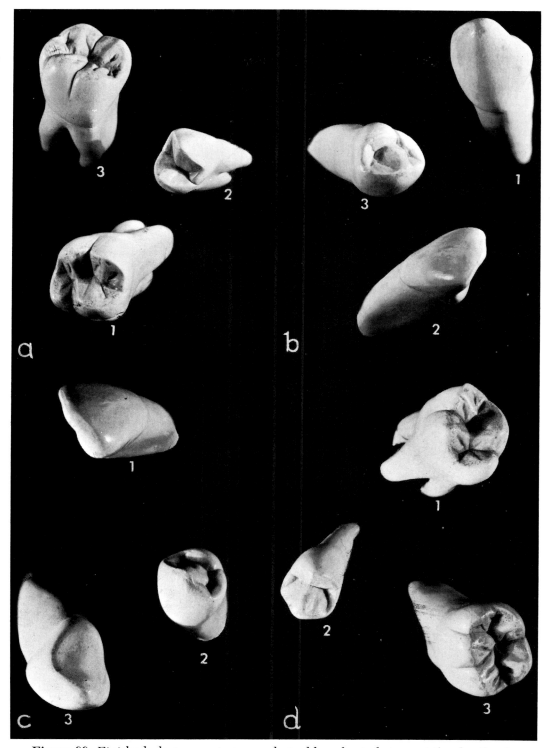

Figure 88. Finished plaster carvings posed at odd angles to bring out the details of tooth form.

    a. 1, Maxillary first molar; 2, maxillary first premolar; 3, mandibular first molar.

    b. 1, Maxillary canine; 2, mandibular canine; 3, mandibular first premolar.

    c. 1, Maxillary central incisor; 2, mandibular first premolar; 3, maxillary canine.

    d. The same teeth illustrated in "*a,*" but at different angulations.

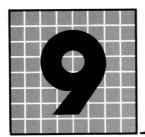

Carving Teeth Normal Size

The plan for blocking in the carvings is the same as shown for plaster sculpture. The procedure is varied to accommodate the use of smaller carving blocks and *the use of measurements in millimeters instead of eighths of an inch*. A flexible millimeter rule, obtainable from a dental supply dealer, is used for marking off the normal size drawings on the blocks; a Boley gauge, to check the calibrations during the various steps in carving.

The complete root form should be included in carvings of teeth normal size. The carvings are complete only when they pass inspection with the caliper and when they have a smooth finish.

The office knife which was used for plaster carving may also be used for the smaller carvings regardless of the material. If hard materials are desired, saws, files or the dental engine may be used to cut away larger sections during the first cuts. More detailed instructions will follow.

Carving blocks may be obtained of hard carving wax (Kerr Dental Mfg. Co., Columbia Dentoform Corp.); a composition imitating tooth dentin (Ivorine, Columbia Dentoform Corp.), or bone. The author has found the material called "Ivorine" to be most satisfactory. It is uniform, of good color and texture, and is molded in sticks of convenient size. The finished carvings take a nice polish and may be safely handled without danger of scarring or breaking when they are set up to study alignment and occlusion.

However, some teachers of tooth carving prefer to use the wax blocks which cut more easily. These blocks have a high melting range and will be preserved under ordinary conditions. Nevertheless, thin sections such as roots are very easily broken, and the texture of the wax which makes it easy to carve also makes it easy to scar in handling. Setting up such carvings in half-jaw arrangement is very difficult.

CARVING IN WAX

Drawings of the teeth to be carved are made on the wax blocks, including the entire root form. A sharp pointed instrument is used to mark the wax. An old dental instrument can be ground for this purpose, or an old-fashioned writing pen with a sharp point is satisfactory.

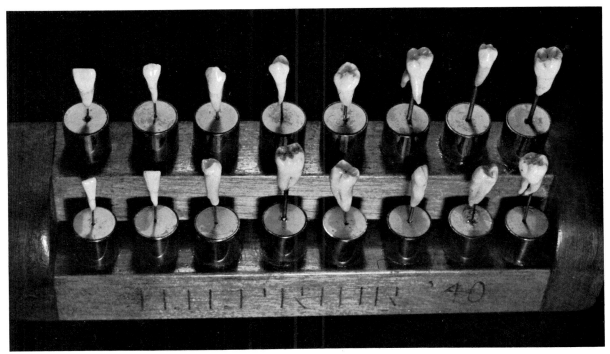

Figure 89. Specimens of human teeth mounted on a stand to be used as models in the study of tooth carving. This ingenious bit of workmanship by a former student made a permanent display for handy reference.

The technique of blocking in and finishing the carving is fundamentally the same as advocated for plaster carving in Chapter 8. The variation lies in the size of the finished carving, the inclusion of the entire root form, and the handling of Ivorine or wax in comparison with plaster. The same meticulous care must be observed in holding to dimensions, accurate calibration during blocking in, and proper technique in finish. The finished carving must include the fundamental tooth form as emphasized in the preceding text.

CARVING IN IVORINE

Ivorine sticks may be procured in three widths to include tooth carvings of varied proportions (Fig. 90).

The outline of the tooth to be carved is drawn on the stick with a sharp pointed lead pencil after sanding the polished surface of the stick slightly to receive the drawing (Fig. 93).

The technique of "blocking in" is observed strictly, just as it was in plaster carving.

Mechanical saws, rasp (vulcanite) files or coarse sand paper discs on a dental engine may be used to cut away the excess beyond the confines of the drawing. Care must be used to avoid frictional heat in the use of rotary discs.

The first carvings on an Ivorine stick may be blocked in on the end of the stick, using the remainder as a convenient holder in the hand or by locking in a bench vise.

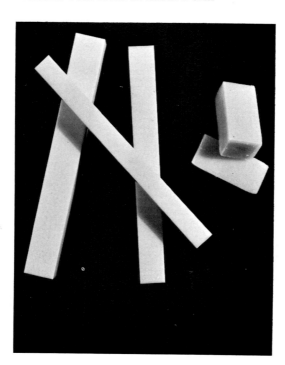

Figure 90. Three sizes of Ivorine sticks and two sizes of carving wax blocks used for carvings (Columbia Dentoform Corp.).

When the blocking in is completed and the calibrations are checked as being correct, the carving is sawed off the stick with a scroll saw.

From this point, the carving may be completed by the exclusive use of a sharp office knife, using a scraping, planing or "pull knife" technique. The straight edge near the point is used for planing off corners and bringing the tooth surfaces down to smooth, curved surfaces within the previously established dimensions. The point of the knife blade and the edge near the point are used only for cutting grooves and depressions in the occlusal surfaces and for outlining cervical lines of the crown (cementoenamel junction) and depressions representing developmental lines and grooves. Most cutting with the point of the blade will be more efficient if a pull stroke is used in dragging the point rather than in an attempt to cut with a push stroke or punching action. Cutting forward with a blade or point is difficult to control and should be avoided whenever possible.

There may be a few occasions in final finishing when it is desirable to obtain a rounded smooth depression obliterating marks left by the point of the knife. The smallest "vulcanite" scraper or a small, sharp, scoop-ended inlay carver will be very satisfactory.

Students who are impatient may be inclined to use burs and discs in a dental engine in attempts to finish carvings more rapidly. *Years of teaching tooth carving have convinced the author that such methods are contraindicated.* Only the most expert carver with years of experience can do it. Inexperienced operators will be unable to control high speed methods. A good sharp office knife properly used on Ivorine will be instrumental in completing a carving smoothly, efficiently, and quickly enough.

The only places where a dental engine is to be used is when removing bulk material beyond drawings on block material. A fissure bur may be used to cut out bulk material between roots when the carving has to show bifurcation. Even in these instances the knife is used as a scraper while finishing the carving.

After the carving is finished so that it is smooth and conforms to anatomic specifications, the dental engine is used to give the carving a final

Text continued on page 107

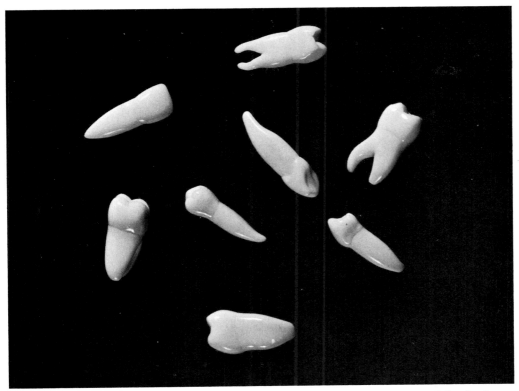

Figure 91. Ivorine carvings by dental students at St. Louis University School of Dentistry.

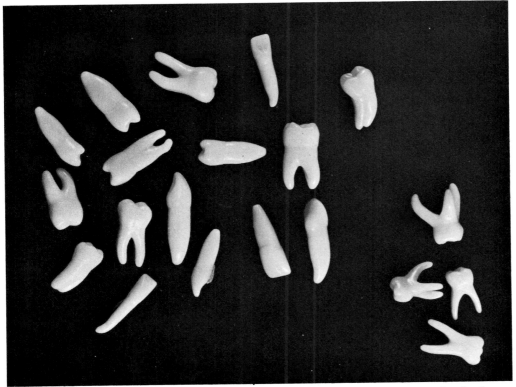

Figure 92. Wax carvings by dental students at Washington University School of Dentistry.

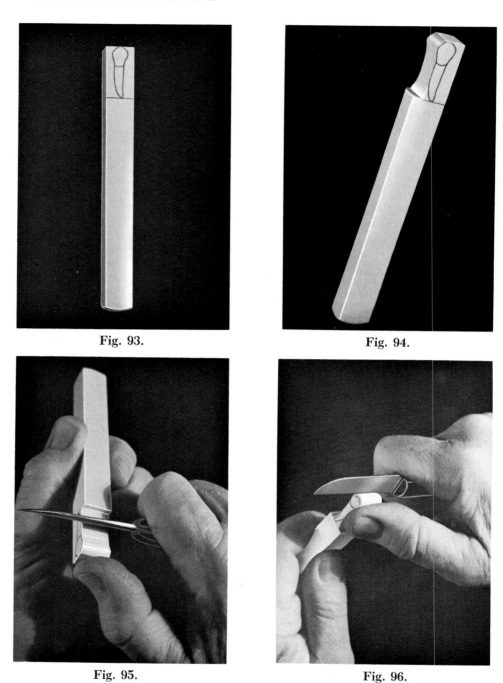

Fig. 93.

Fig. 94.

Fig. 95.

Fig. 96.

Figure 93. Ivorine stick with drawing of carving to be made. The outline is drawn in reverse on the opposite side.

Figure 94. One side has been cut away and planed down to outline. The first cut is complete.

Figure 95. Same as Figure 94 showing application of knife and relation of blade to carving. The knife is being used as a plane. A "draw knife" technique is used, with the center of the blade in contact with the carving.

Figure 96. The second cut being completed.

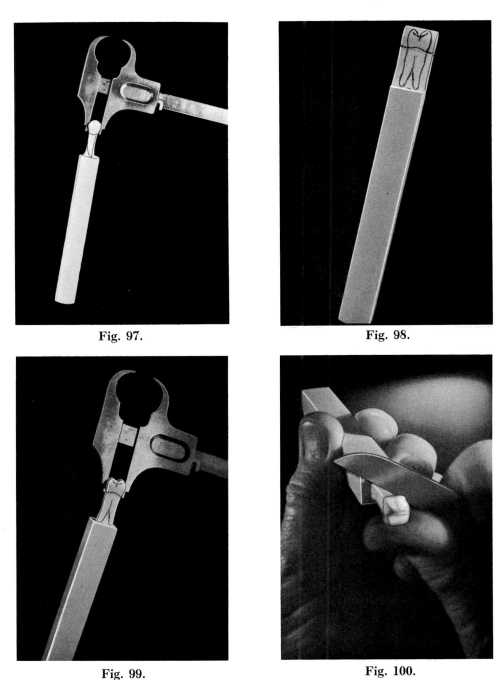

Fig. 97.   Fig. 98.

Fig. 99.   Fig. 100.

Figure 97. Checking the measurement after the completion of two cuts.

Figure 98. Buccolingual drawing to be followed in making the third and fourth cuts.

Figure 99. Calibrating after the fourth cut; blocking in has been completed.

Figure 100. Rounding the first corner of the blocked-in carving.

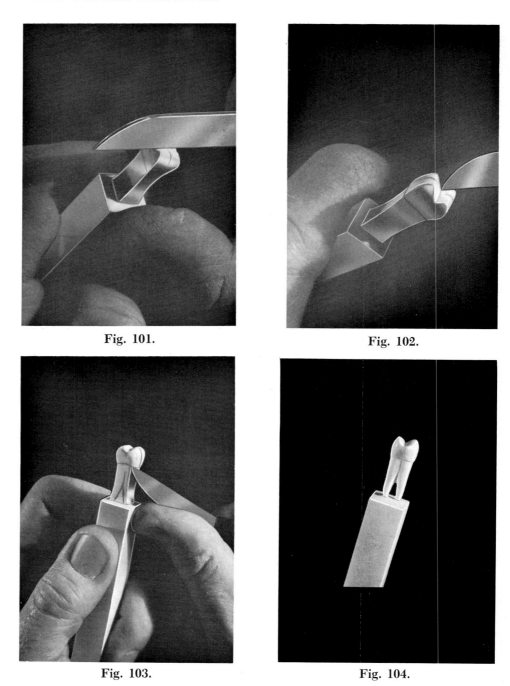

Fig. 101.   Fig. 102.

Fig. 103.   Fig. 104.

Figure 101. Sulcus of occlusal surface has been notched level with future marginal ridges. (See Fig. 84.)

Figure 102. Position of blade while planing occlusal incline.

Figure 103. Outlining the cervix by engraving with knife edge close to point. (See Fig. 83.)

Figure 104. Finished carving of the maxillary first premolar.

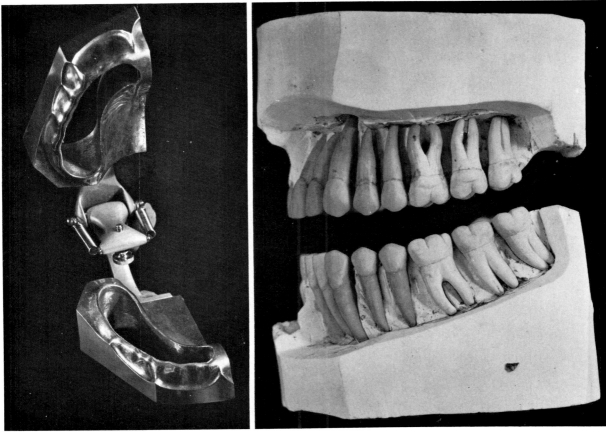

Fig. 105.   Fig. 106.

Figure 105. Half-jaw articulator made with cells to accommodate wax for the set-up of complete carvings (Columbia Dentoform Corp.).

Figure 106. Original set up of carvings by the author with plaster bases dissected. This shows the angulation of roots in the alignment of carvings in centric relation.

polish. Small brush wheels (prophylactic brush wheels) dipped in flour of pumice and water are used in the dental engine to give the carving its final polish, using care not to cut or scratch the surface by high speed or by holding the brush on one spot too long. When scratches have been removed by this method and the carving has a dull polish, a very high polish may be obtained by rotating the carving against a soft rag wheel on a bench lathe, using a paste of chalk and water. The rag wheel must be very soft and the carving must be rotated against it with very light pressure.

When the normal size carvings are completed they are to be "set up" in centric occlusion in a half-jaw articulator designed for the purpose (Figs. 105 to 108).

Modeling clay is placed in the bottom of the wells and the apices of the roots of the teeth are imbedded in it to hold each tooth in place until alignment and occlusion of the teeth have been accomplished. No more than one-half of the root should be covered by the clay.

When the teeth are in their proper relationship to each other, pink base plate wax is melted and poured into the wells around the teeth, fixing them in position. After the wax has cooled (care must be used not to pour

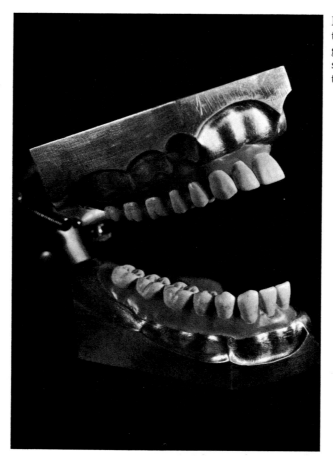

Figure 107. Completed tooth carvings set up in good alignment and occlusion in the special articulator.

Figure 108. Half-jaw set up of carvings in the articulator — closed in centric relation.

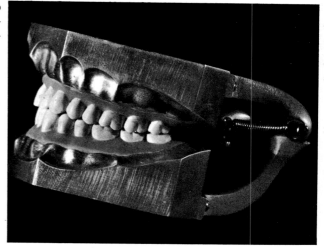

the wax too hot) the modeling clay may be picked out from the bottom of the wells and replaced with plaster of Paris. This fixes the roots in position. If wax is used for this purpose also, the great bulk of wax may cause the teeth to warp out of alignment.

If the wax is poured just level with the wells in the articulator, the crowns of the teeth and the cervical portion of the roots will remain exposed. Additional pink base plate wax is now applied with a wax spatula, built up and festooned to simulate gingival tissue around the teeth (Figs. 107 and 108).

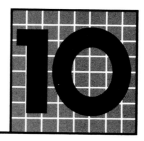

Illustrations To Be Used
for Reference Purposes
in Carving

For the purpose of our discussion of the subject of tooth form and its attendant details, it can be said that since restorative work in dentistry is a manual art which must approach the scientific as closely as manual dexterity will allow, models, plans, photographs and anatomic specimens should be given preference over the written text. Visual aids, especially those exhibiting three dimensional figures, are of inestimable value in the study of form.

On the following pages, drawings of the eight typal tooth forms may be used for reference. Also enlarged photographs of specimen teeth may be consulted.

	Page Numbers for Typal Forms	*Page Numbers for Specimen Teeth*
Maxillary teeth	Central incisor 110	Central incisor 111
		Lateral incisor 111
	Canine 112	Canine 113
	First premolar 114	First premolar 115
		Second premolar 115
	First molar 116	First molar 117
		Second molar 117
Mandibular teeth	Central incisor 118	Central incisor 119
		Lateral incisor 119
	Canine 120	Canine 121
	First premolar 122	First premolar 123
		Second premolar 123
	First molar 124	First molar 125
		Second molar 125

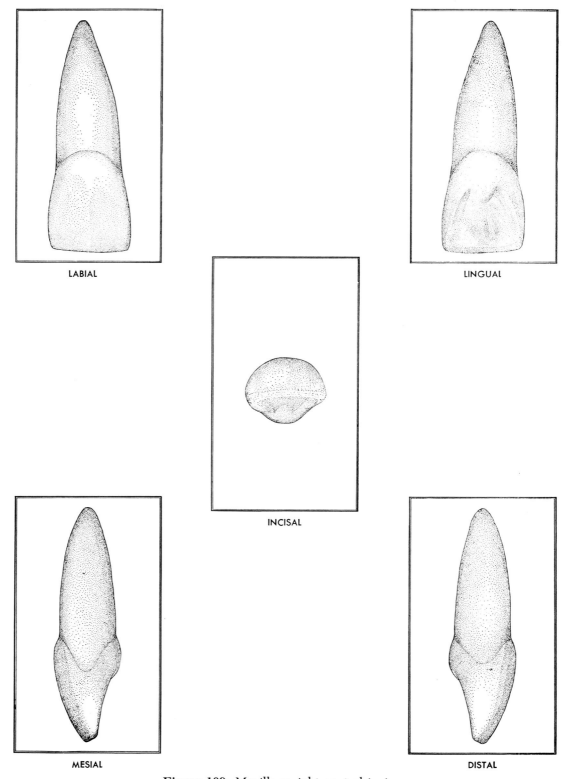

LABIAL

LINGUAL

INCISAL

MESIAL

DISTAL

Figure 109. Maxillary right central incisor.

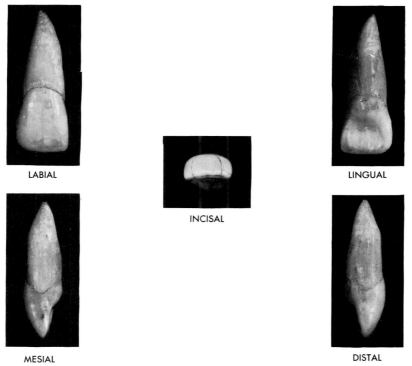

Figure 110. Maxillary right central incisor.

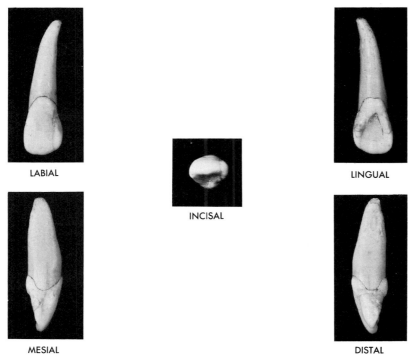

Figure 111. Maxillary left lateral incisor.

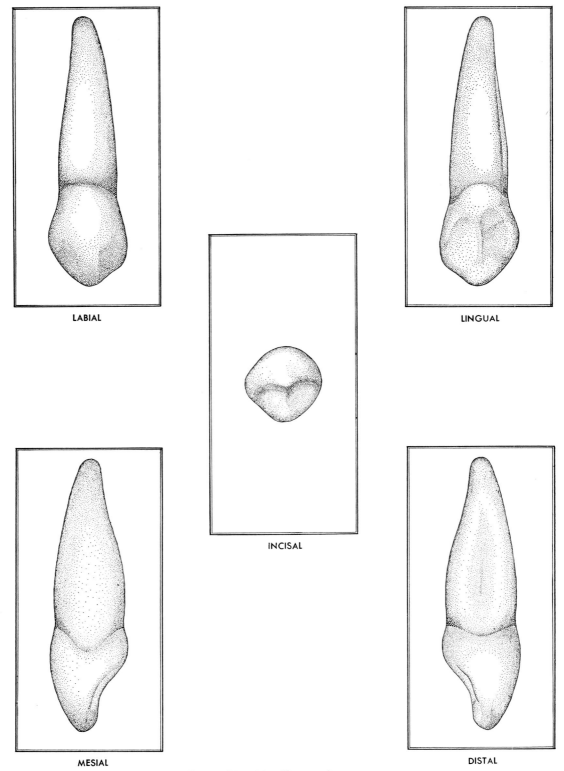

Figure 112. Maxillary right canine.

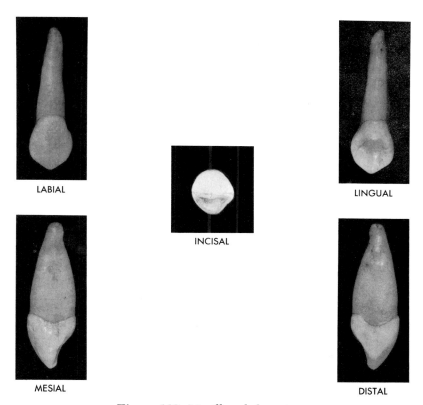

LABIAL

INCISAL

LINGUAL

MESIAL

DISTAL

Figure 113. Maxillary left canine.

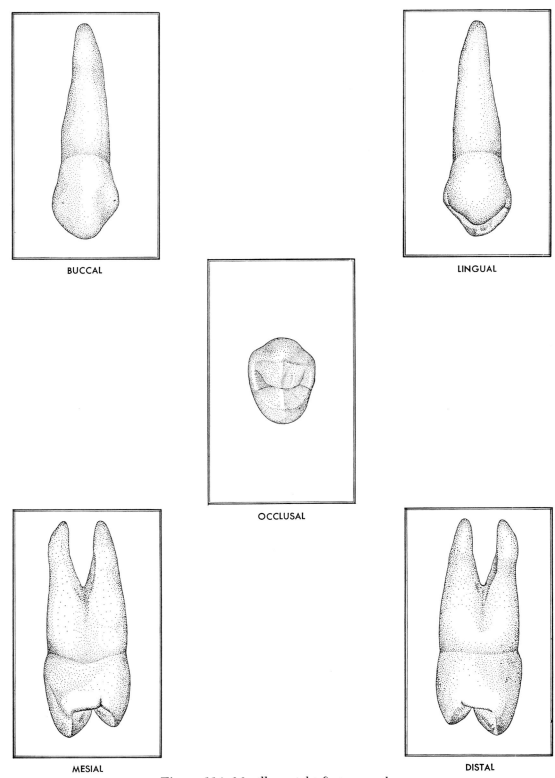

BUCCAL

LINGUAL

OCCLUSAL

MESIAL

DISTAL

Figure 114. Maxillary right first premolar.

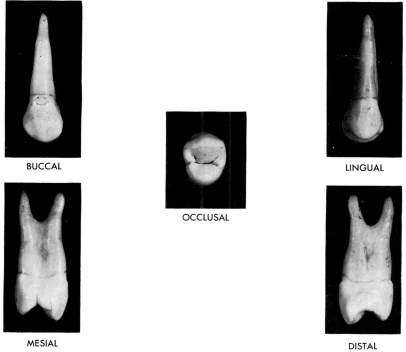

BUCCAL

OCCLUSAL

LINGUAL

MESIAL

DISTAL

Figure 115. Maxillary left first premolar.

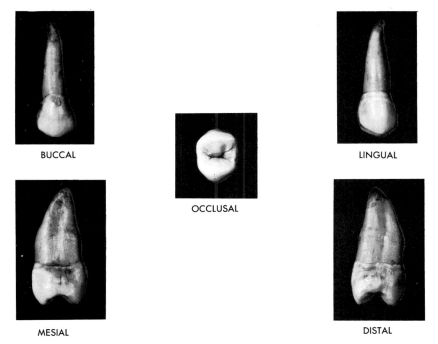

BUCCAL

OCCLUSAL

LINGUAL

MESIAL

DISTAL

Figure 116. Maxillary left second premolar.

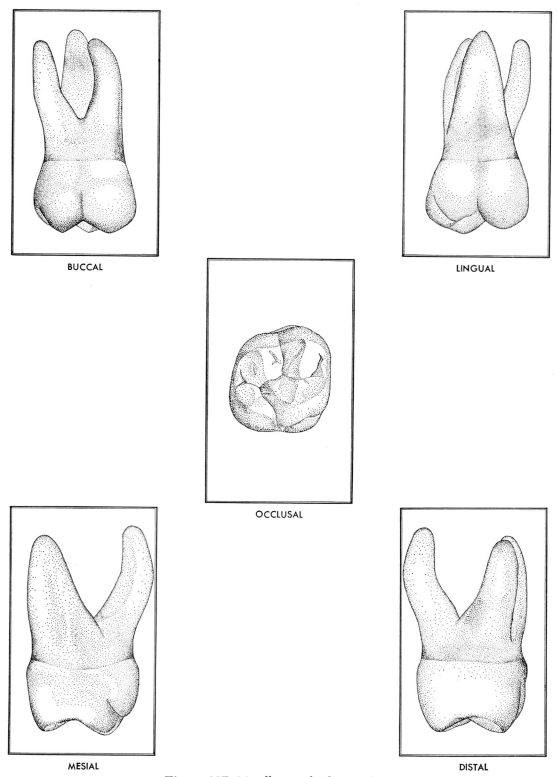

BUCCAL

LINGUAL

OCCLUSAL

MESIAL

DISTAL

Figure 117. Maxillary right first molar.

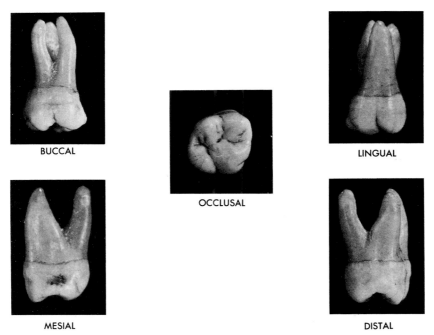

Figure 118. Maxillary right first molar.

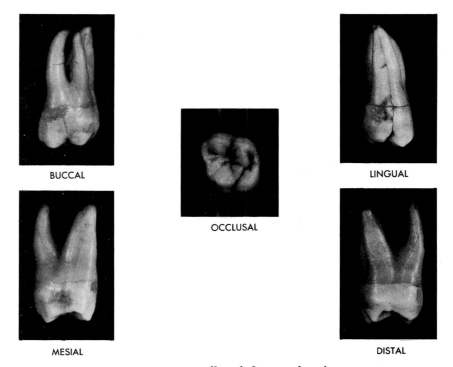

Figure 119. Maxillary left second molar.

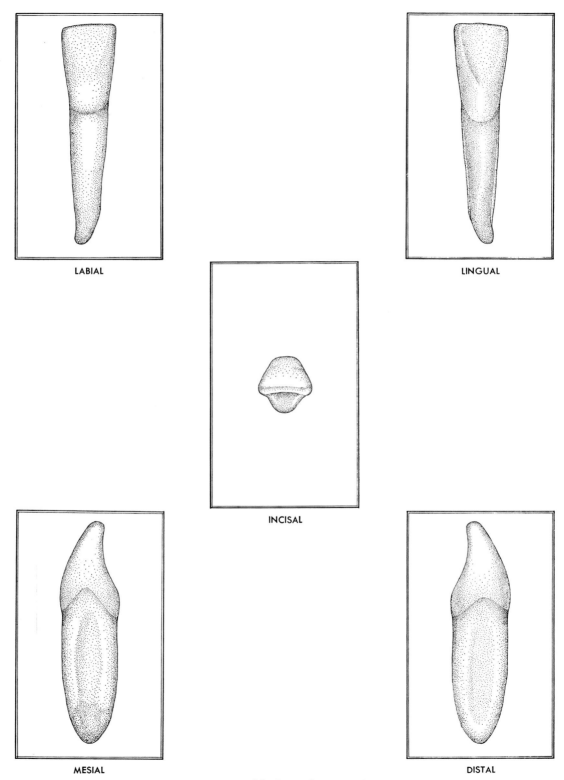

LABIAL

LINGUAL

INCISAL

MESIAL

DISTAL

Figure 120. Mandibular right central incisor.

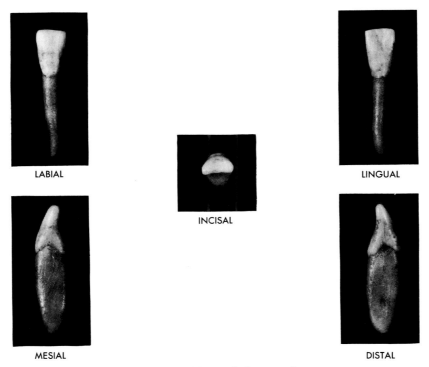

Figure 121. Mandibular left central incisor.

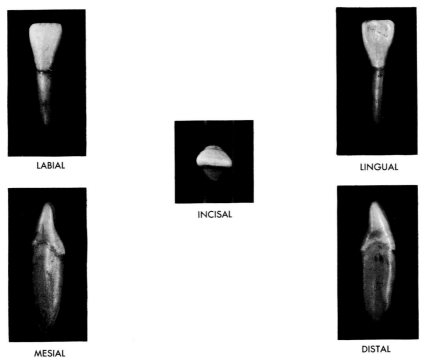

Figure 122. Mandibular right lateral incisor.

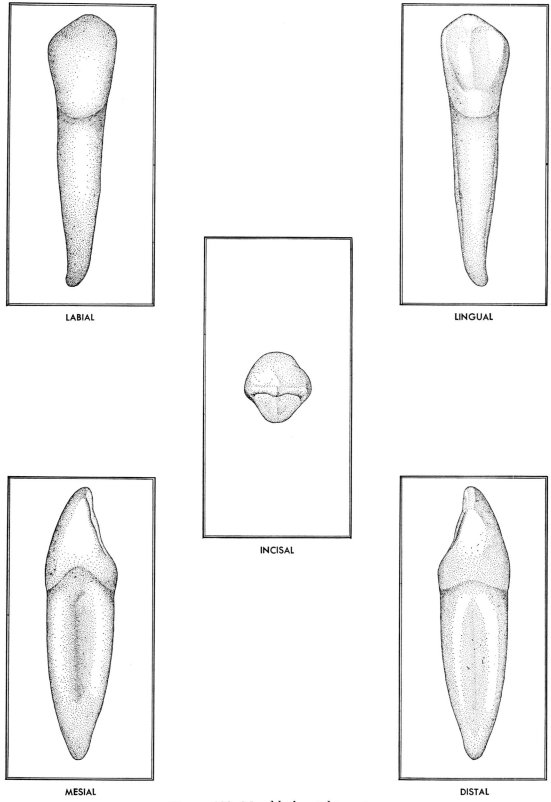

LABIAL

LINGUAL

INCISAL

MESIAL

DISTAL

Figure 123. Mandibular right canine.

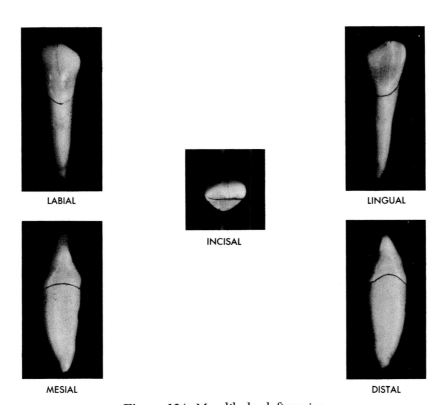

Figure 124. Mandibular left canine.

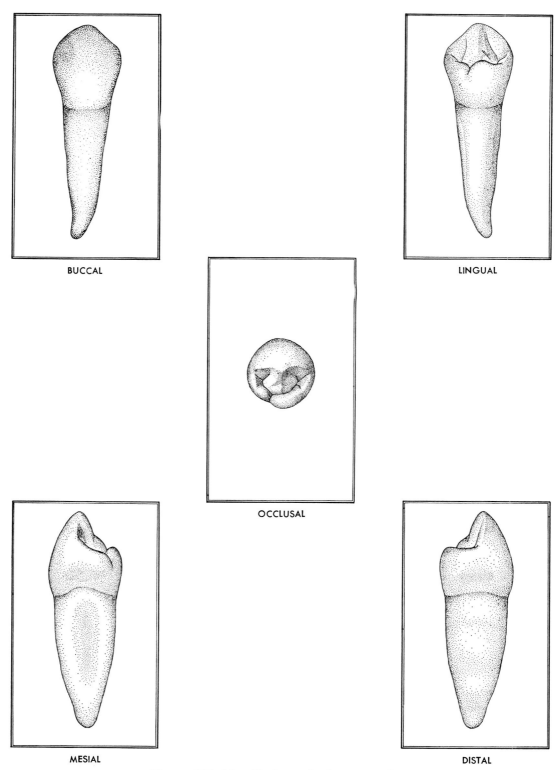

BUCCAL

LINGUAL

OCCLUSAL

MESIAL

DISTAL

Figure 125. Mandibular right first premolar.

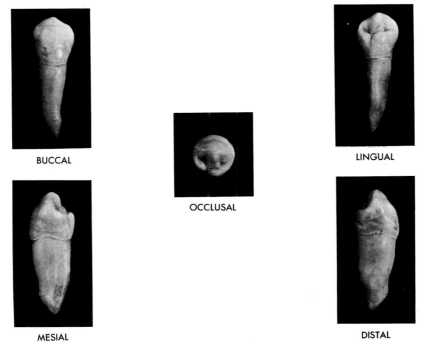

BUCCAL OCCLUSAL LINGUAL

MESIAL DISTAL

Figure 126. Mandibular right first premolar.

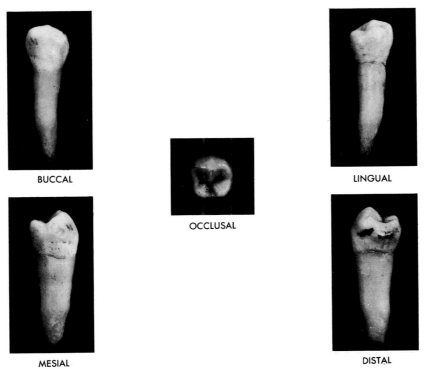

BUCCAL OCCLUSAL LINGUAL

MESIAL DISTAL

Figure 127. Mandibular left second premolar.

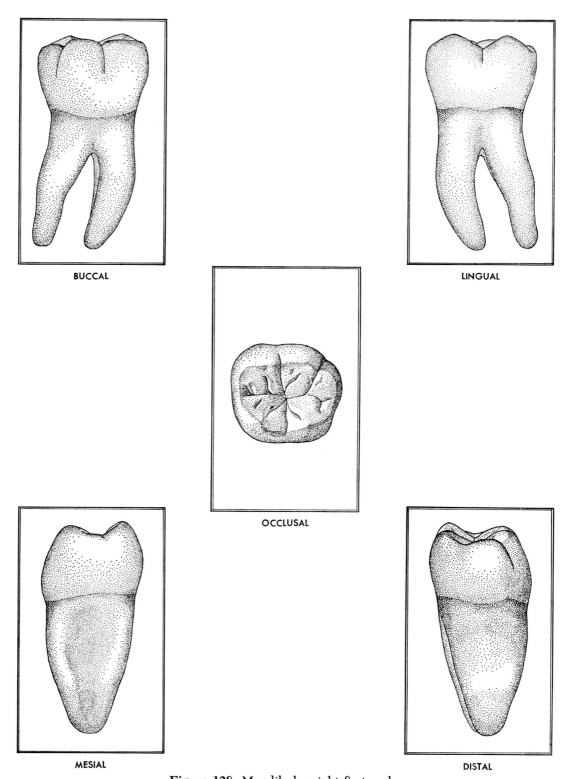

BUCCAL

LINGUAL

OCCLUSAL

MESIAL

DISTAL

Figure 128. Mandibular right first molar.

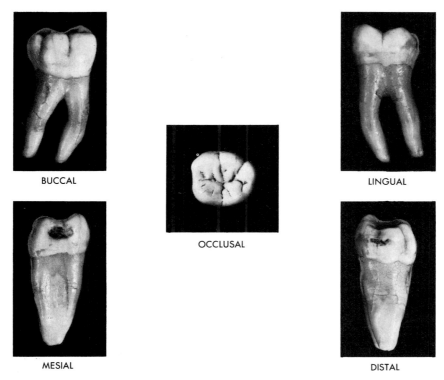

BUCCAL

OCCLUSAL

LINGUAL

MESIAL

DISTAL

Figure 129. Mandibular right first molar.

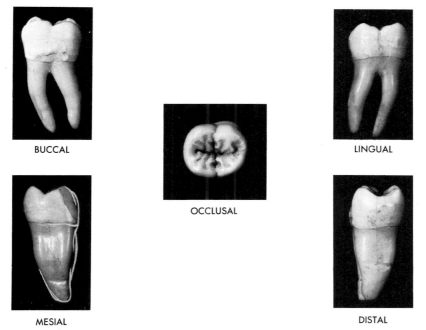

BUCCAL

OCCLUSAL

LINGUAL

MESIAL

DISTAL

Figure 130. Mandibular left second molar.

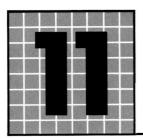

Arrangement of the Teeth and Occlusion

The teeth are arranged in two opposing series; one is fixed (maxillary series), and the other is movable (mandibular series). Each series is made up of 16 components (counting third molars) arranged so that they form a dental arch (Fig. 131).

The mandibular arch which is movable operates against the maxillary arch which is fixed during functional jaw movements. Students of dental physiology (and many dentists, for that matter) are inclined to forget on occasion that this situation exists. The reason for the temporary aberration is this: Mechanical dental articulators used in the laboratory for dental prosthesis have the maxillary member movable with the mandibular member fixed, which is just the opposite arrangement from that found in the human jaws. Mechanically, the dental articulator design simplifies the instrument for practical use in the laboratory. Nevertheless, it may influence the operator's thinking unless he is careful to keep reminding himself of the true relation of the jaws.

It is most important in the study of occlusion to realize that the primary forces of occlusion are brought to bear upon the immovable maxillary arch by the movable mandibular arch.

There are five positions of the mandible that are usually described: centric relation, centric occlusion, right and left lateral, and protrusive. These are occlusal relations. Centric relation is a jaw-to-jaw relationship with the condyles in their midmost, uppermost position. Centric relation may be coincident with centric occlusion in which there is considered to be the intercuspal position of the teeth. Centric occlusion is anterior to centric relation in the majority of natural dentitions.

The most important of these is *centric occlusion*. In *centric occlusion* there is an intercusping relation between all the posterior teeth of both arches on both right and left sides. At the same time all the anterior teeth of one arch are in contact with those of the other arch.

In *centric occlusion* lines of force brought to bear upon the fixed base or maxillary arch by the movable or mandibular arch are equalized and absorbed by the mutual aid of all the teeth. The entire dental mechanism is designed to cooperate with the design of, and to achieve finally, centric occlusion as the ultimate terminal in function.

In order to bring about right and left lateral relations in occlusion and protrusive relation, the temporomandibular joint allows intricate movements and changing points of rotation in order to compensate for the various positions.

There will be no attempt made in this Atlas to describe all the intricacies of tooth arrangement and occlusion which involve temporomandibular articulation and the more involved occlusal relations. That is a specialized subject which must be studied in a more advanced course and with a more complete textbook.

FUNCTIONAL FORM OF THE TEETH AT THEIR INCISAL AND OCCLUSAL THIRDS

First, it will be well to reconsider the functional form of the teeth at their incisal and occlusal thirds (Figs. 132 and 133). Note also the angulation of the axes in centric relation. The anterior teeth in these illustrations are inclined labially so that their axis inclination is 30 degrees to the vertical at the minimum angulation. The maxillary teeth extend labially over the mandibular teeth. The curved incisal edges of the mandibular incisors will contact the maxillary incisors on their concave lingual surfaces above the incisal ridges. This arrangement allows a certain degree of *overbite* and *overjet*, which will vary with individuals.

Vertical overlap (overbite) is that characteristic of the teeth in which the incisal ridges of the maxillary anterior teeth extend below the incisal ridges of the mandibular teeth when the jaws are closed.

Horizontal overlap (overjet) is that characteristic of all the maxillary teeth to extend facially beyond the contours of the mandibular teeth.

When discussing the alignment or "set-up" of teeth we speak of the relative degree of vertical or horizontal overlap (Figs. 134, 135).

Figure 132 shows the angle at which anterior and posterior crowns are set in order to approach centric relation. Note also that posterior teeth (premolars and molars) have the buccal cusps of mandibular teeth contacting central sulci of maxillary teeth. Lingual cusps of maxillary teeth contact central sulci of mandibular teeth. The tips of buccal cusps of maxillary teeth are out of contact in centric and the tips of lingual cusps of mandibular teeth are out of contact. This arrangement serves to confine the shock or forces of contact within the root bases of these teeth. In short, the lines of force in centric are parallel or confluent with the long axes of the posterior teeth whether they are maxillary or mandibular.

The main bulk of the tooth crowns of mandibular posterior teeth is made up of the buccal cusps leaning lingually in order to be more centered over the root base. The lingual cusps increase the "food table" but normally are out of contact during all occlusal relations. The mandibular posterior teeth are the active (movable) ones, of course, and at the time of closure of the jaws they operate as cutters or grinders as they contact the immovable maxillary posterior teeth in the centric portion of the "food table" between the cusps of maxillary posterior teeth (Fig. 136).

By this time the student should realize that *there are no flat surfaces or planes to be found on normal teeth except those that are present due to wear or accident.* Plane surfaces would not allow escapement, would put greater stress upon tissue attachment, and would not allow any variation in tooth arrangement. The normal curved surfaces are more efficient in cutting

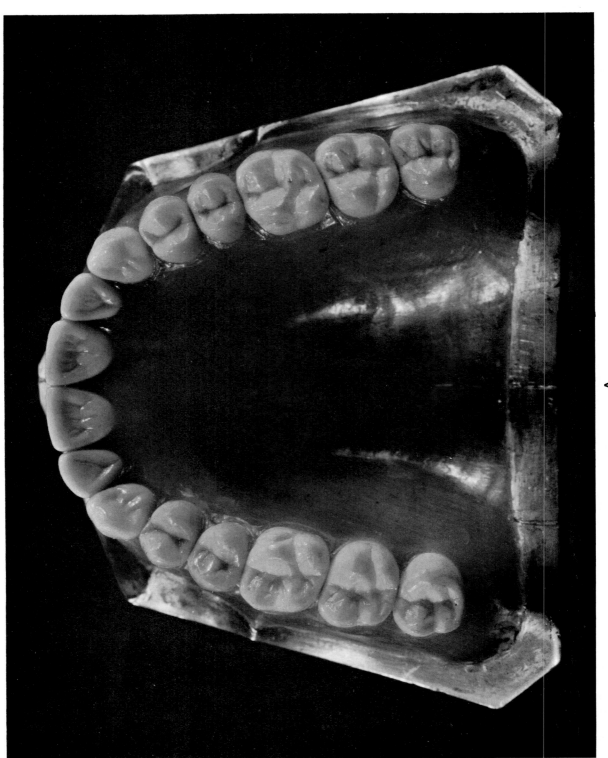

A

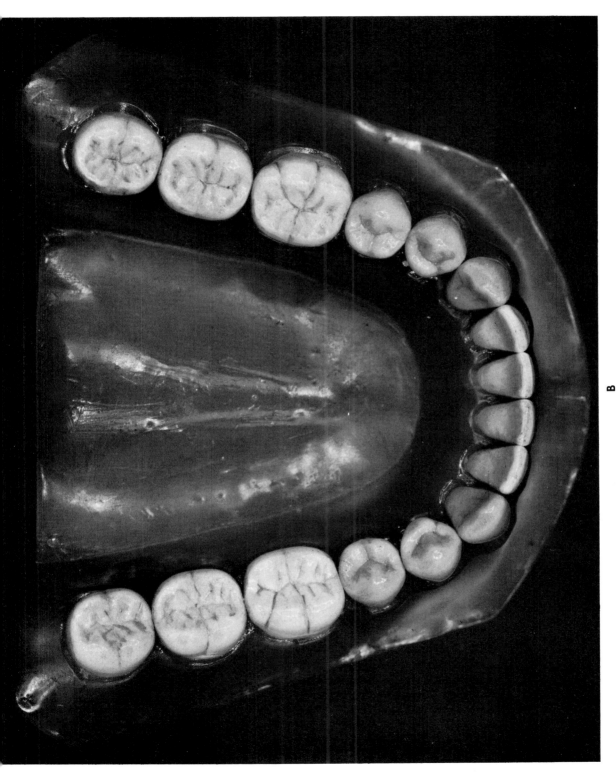

B

Figure 131. Model teeth carved by the author and placed in "ideal" alignment and contact relation. *A,* Maxillary arch; *B,* mandibular arch. See Figures 29 and 30.

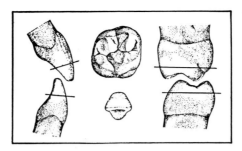

Figure 132. Functional form of the teeth at their incisal and occlusal thirds.

Figure 133. The incisal or occlusal thirds of the tooth crowns present convex or concave surfaces at all contacting occlusal areas.

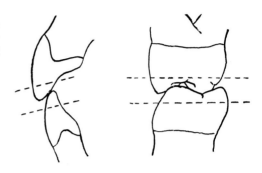

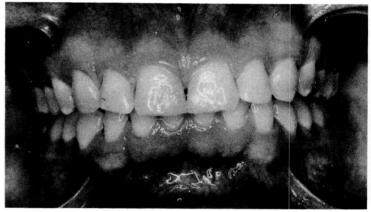

Figure 134. Demonstration of vertical and horizontal overlays.

Figure 135. Overbite and overjet. (Graber: Textbook of Orthodontics.)

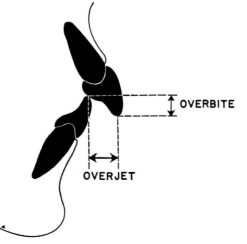

Figure 136. The cycle of occlusal movements, represented by a schematic drawing of first molar relations — mesial aspect. The heavy outline of the mandibular molar represents it in centric occlusal relation to the maxillary molar. The shadow outlines represent the mandibular molar in various relations during the cycle of manidbular movement during mastication. The two short lines at right angles to the occlusal surface of the maxillary molar measure the extent of movement over the occlusal surface from the first contact of the mandibular molar to the last contact before continuing another cycle.

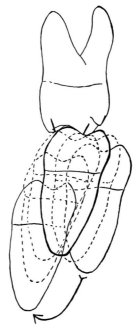

food material, allowing escapement where there is no contact around and about the crests of curvature as they come together.

The curved surfaces of occlusal and incisal portions of the tooth crowns give the entire dental mechanism a definite advantage in stability. It is possible to have great efficiency even when the alignment of individual teeth is not ideal, and of course ideal alignment is seldom found. Flat planes to be efficient would require that opposing teeth be in one position only, so that opposing planes might become parallel on contact. On contact, the lack of spacing for escapement would increase the force on root bases tremendously.

DENTAL ARCH FORMATION (ALIGNMENT)

The dental arch forms are illustrated in Figures 131 and 137.

In the optimum functional arrangement of the teeth the arches are balanced bilaterally on each side of the median plane.

The arch form may be broken down into three segments: anterior, middle and posterior segments. These segments are described by the curvature or direction or inclination of the labial and buccal surfaces. Actually, since the teeth are in close contact relation, there is an overlapping of the teeth of one segment with those of the next.

The anterior segment of the maxillary arch is made up of the anterior teeth, including the mesial half of the canine; the middle segment includes the distal half of the canine, the two premolars and the mesial third of the first molar; the posterior segment includes the distal two-thirds of the first molar and the second and third molars. The crests of contour labially and buccally will describe a smooth curved outline to the anterior segment, but straight lines will describe the alignment of the middle and posterior segments.

The anterior segment of the mandibular arch will show even curvature to the crest of contour of the canine; a straight line for the middle segment,

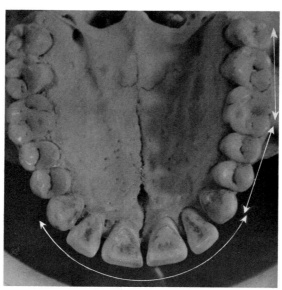

Figure 137. A photograph of the dental arches of a natural specimen. The white lines show the approximate alignment in segments of the labial and buccal surfaces of the dental arches.

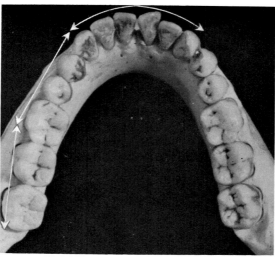

including the distal half of the canine, the premolars and the mesial two-thirds of the first molar; the posterior segment, a straight line from the distobuccal cusp of the first molar parallel with the buccal surfaces of the second and third molars.

COMPENSATING CURVATURE OF THE DENTAL ARCHES

In order to achieve "balance" during the various mandibular movements, the axes of the teeth are arranged so that the incisal and occlusal surfaces of both arches adapt themselves to curved planes. Compensating occlusal curvature is a subject too vast to be covered in this work. However, the student must be aware of the truism that this principle exists. The normal arrangement of teeth will not permit proper function if incisal and occlusal surfaces adapt themselves to a rigidly flat plane.

Observation of Figures 138 and 139 will show actual examples of the curvature; one is a photograph of a human skull, and the other is a cast from an impression of a living person.

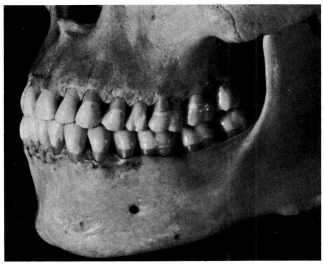

Figure 138. Centric occlusion. This illustration shows normal occlusion. Note the compensating curvature of the occlusal thirds of all the teeth. (Draw a line following the incisal ridges and cusp tips of the maxillary teeth.) Also note the margin of the alveolar process in its relation to the cervical line of the teeth.

CONTACT RELATIONS OF THE TEETH

Of particular importance is the contact relations of the opposing teeth in centric occlusion. The contacts of supporting cusps (mandibular buccal cusps and maxillary lingual cusps) with opposing fossae or marginal ridges are called *centric stops* (Figs. 139, 140). In a normal occlusion there are contact relations in lateral excursions (Fig. 141). The cuspid may or not provide disclusion of posterior teeth.

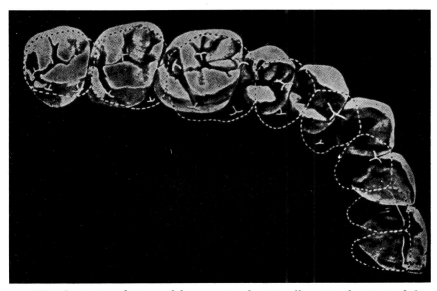

Figure 139. Contact relation of human teeth. Maxillary teeth. Dotted lines of mandibular teeth superposed in occlusion. (Courtesy of Sheldon Freil, Dublin.)

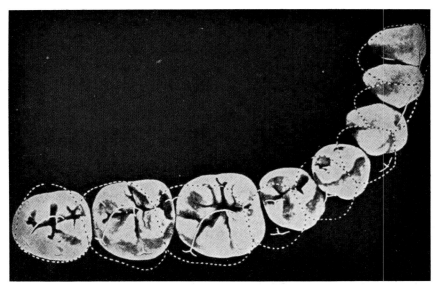

Figure 140. Contact relation of human teeth. Mandibular teeth. Dotted lines of maxillary teeth superposed in occlusion. (Courtesy of Sheldon Freil, Dublin.)

Each tooth in each arch has two antagonists in the opposing arch, except the mandibular central incisor and the maxillary third molar. In the event of the loss of any tooth, this arrangement tends to prevent extrusion of antagonists and helps to stabilize the remaining teeth over a longer period than would be likely if each tooth had a single antagonist. (See Fig. 13.)

Figure 141. Occlusal contacts made in right lateral movement with "normal" arrangement of teeth. *A*, Maxillary teeth. *B*, Mandibular teeth.

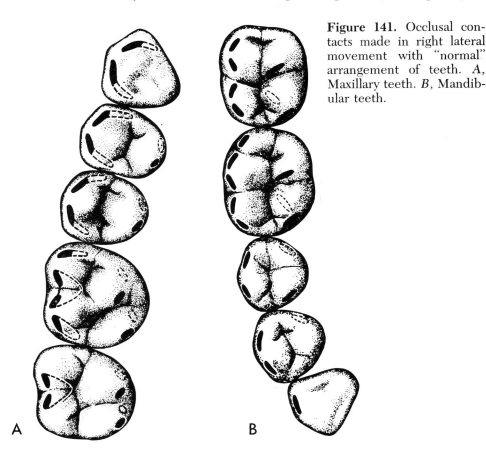

A   B

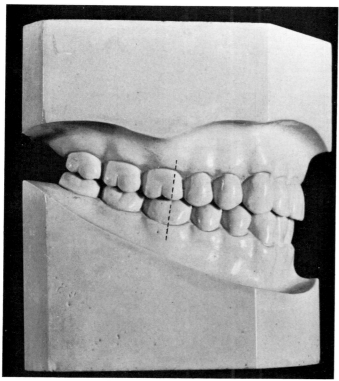

Figure 142. Normal occlusion and alignment in centric relation from the buccal aspect directly opposite the first molars. The relationship of first molars is the "key of occlusion." Note the relationship of the mesiobuccal cusp of the maxillary molar to the mesiobuccal developmental groove of the mandibular molar.

OCCLUSAL CONTACT AND INTERCUSP RELATIONS

A study of the occlusal contact of opposing teeth in centric occlusal relation will emphasize basic points as follows:

The mesial surfaces of central incisors, both maxillary and mandibular, are placed at the median line.

The mandibular central incisor, because it is narrow distally, will contact the maxillary central only.

Every other tooth, both maxillary and mandibular, will show contact with two opposing teeth except the most posterior maxillary tooth, which in a full complement is the third molar (Figs. 139, 140).

When studying the offset arrangement of the alignment (one against two), note particularly that, in most instances, the teeth are not centered like bricks in a wall where one brick is bisected by the contact of the two opposing ones. Rather, each tooth of one arch contacts less than half of one opponent and more than half of another. In fact, the molars are offset very little. This arrangement is made possible by varying mesiodistal measurements.

The highest points of major ridges and cusps are located in Figures 139 and 140 with heavy marked *lines* or *T's* to show their relations with opposing teeth when the jaws are closed and the teeth of both dental arches are in centric relation.

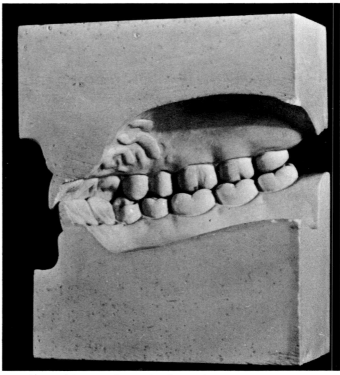

Figure 143. Centric occlusion from the lingual aspect. Another view of the casts shown in Figure 142.

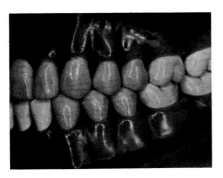

Figure 144. Labiobuccal aspect of the teeth in centric occlusion. This aspect is taken from a position directly in line with the labial surface of the maxillary canine.

Figure 145. Buccal aspect of the teeth in centric occlusion. This aspect is taken from a position directly buccal to the mesiobuccal cusp of the maxillary first molar.

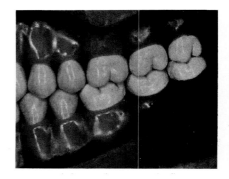

When the jaws come together and the teeth are in this relationship, the jaw force is equalized so that the individual tooth, assisted by the combined resistance of all of them, is best able to withstand the force and remain stable.

Another important observation is this: In only one location will a cusp be found contacting the opposing teeth directly above the contact areas. In that instance it is the mesiobuccal cusp of the mandibular first molar, which approaches the contact relation to the maxillary second premolar and first molar in centric relation.

However, the mesiobuccal cusp of the mandibular first molar is broad and flat in comparison with sharper cusps of some other teeth. In addition, the roll of marginal ridges allows space for escapement. At every other point the plan seems to be to avoid a sharp cusp directly against contacting members which might act as a wedge, forcing food material between the teeth. Also, the cusps would be less efficient as cutters if they did not contact a broader, solid surface.

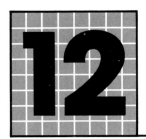

The Deciduous Teeth

As the term "deciduous" implies, these teeth are shed in order to make way for their permanent successors.* Only the form of the deciduous teeth will be covered in this publication. Further information concerning the anatomy and physiology of deciduous teeth and their development will be found in a complete textbook of dental anatomy (Dental Anatomy, Physiology and Occlusion, W. B. Saunders Company). Figure 146 and Figure 147, A and B, will illustrate a normal deciduous dentition and will identify the individual teeth. There are no premolars and no third molars.

There will be no attempt to describe the tooth form of deciduous teeth in this book in as much detail (and that includes illustrations) as was done with the permanent dentition. Since the primary object of the Atlas is to foster the accurate and physiologic restoration of teeth, more consideration must be given to the permanent teeth.

Restoration of deciduous teeth, although very necessary at times, may be handled with less effort than restoration of permanent teeth because rapid changes in development while the deciduous teeth are being used make most details in curvature inoperative as a requirement for permanency. Figure 147 shows casts from a child five and one-half years old. The jaw development only three years after the arch was complete has caused such expansion of the arch that the teeth have separated. The interproximal and contact area form and the original occlusal form are not functioning according to the rules laid down for the normal form and arrangement for permanent teeth. Yet observation of the mouths of developing children will show that the soft tissue is normal when this condition exists and that the children suffer no ill effects.

Periodontal reactions to irritation are certainly not the same in children as those experienced by adults. Restorations showing less finesse in reproduction will be tolerated in the child's mouth, but work that is crude and unhygienic must be avoided.

---

*The term "primary dentition" has been accepted as preferable to the term "deciduous dentition" by the Terminology Committee of the American Society of Dentistry for Children. Among all other interested groups, however, the first set of teeth is termed "deciduous" rather than "primary."

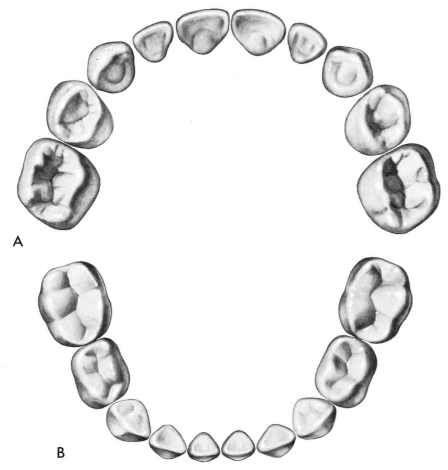

Figure 146. The primary dentition.

Apparently the deciduous teeth have been well designed for their purposes; although their individual form does not change with the growing foundation tissues, they manage to function very well as masticatory tools, even though the jaws are expanding rapidly and the permanent teeth are developing within them. The importance of the deciduous teeth must not be discounted; some of them are in use for 11 years or more, during some

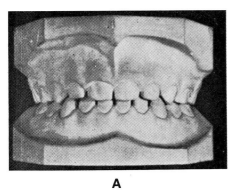
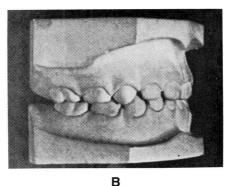

A   **B**

Figure 147. Casts of normally developed teeth of a child five and a half years old. Note the form and occlusion of the teeth and their even separation. *A*, Labial aspect; *B*, buccal aspect. Occlusal aspects of these teeth are shown in Figure 146. (Courtesy Columbia Dentoform Co., New York.)

years of great physical change. Undoubtedly if the deciduous teeth can continue to function until the proper time for their exfoliation, they will assist materially in jaw development in addition to performing their daily duties in contributing to the child's health and welfare.

DESCRIPTION OF THE DECIDUOUS TEETH

Incisors and Canines

Labial Aspects—Maxillary (Fig. 148 a, b, c)

In the crown of the deciduous incisors the mesiodistal diameter is greater than the cervicoincisal length. (The opposite situation exists in permanent incisors.) The labial surfaces are very smooth and the incisal edges are nearly straight. Developmental lines are usually not seen. The roots are cone-shaped with evenly tapered sides. The root lengths are greater in comparison to the crown lengths than in the permanent incisors. It will be well in studying the deciduous teeth to make direct comparisons between the table of measurements of the deciduous teeth and the table of measurements for the permanent teeth (page 26 and page 141).

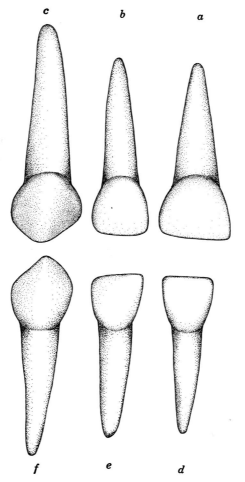

Figure 148. Deciduous right anterior teeth, labial aspect. *a,* Maxillary central incisor; *b,* maxillary lateral incisor; *c,* maxillary canine; *d,* mandibular central incisor; *e,* mandibular lateral incisor; *f,* mandibular canine.

Table 2. Table of Measurements of the Deciduous Teeth of Man (G. V. Black) (Averages Only)

	Length Over All	Length of Crown	Length of Root	Mesio-distal Diameter of Crown	Mesio-distal Diameter at Cervix	Labio-lingual Diameter of Crown	Labio-lingual Diameter at Cervix
Maxillary Teeth							
Central Incisor	16.0*	6.0	10.0	6.5	4.5	5.0	4.0
Lateral Incisor	15.8	5.6	11.4	5.1	3.7	4.8	3.7
Canine	19.0	6.5	13.5	7.0	5.1	7.0	5.5
First Molar	15.2	5.1	10.0	7.3	5.2	8.5	6.9
Second Molar	17.5	5.7	11.7	8.2	6.4	10.0	8.3
Mandibular Teeth							
Central Incisor	14.0	5.0	9.0	4.2	3.0	4.0	3.5
Lateral Incisor	15.0	5.2	10.0	4.1†	3.0	4.0	3.5
Canine	17.0	6.0	11.5	5.0	3.7	4.8	4.0
First Molar	15.8	6.0	9.8	7.7	6.5	7.0	5.3
Second Molar	18.8	5.5	11.3	9.9	7.2	8.7	6.4

*Millimeters.

†This measurement should be greater, approximately the same as the mandibular central incisor. (R. C. W.)

Except for the root form, the labial aspect of the maxillary canine does not resemble either maxillary incisor. The crown is more constricted at the cervix in relation to mesiodistal width, and the mesial and distal surfaces are more convex. Instead of an incisal edge, relatively straight, it has a long, well-developed cusp.

The cusp on the deciduous canine is longer and sharper than that of the permanent maxillary canine, and the contact areas are level with each other, their levels being about half the distance from cervical line labially to cusp tip. Contact areas are not at the same level on permanent canines.

The root of the deciduous canine is very long compared to crown length.

Labial Aspects—Mandibular (Fig. 148 d, e, f)

The labial surfaces of deciduous mandibular incisors are smooth and flat with no developmental markings. The mesial and distal sides of the crowns are tapered evenly from the contact areas, the measurement at the cervix being quite narrow when compared to the measurement at the contact levels. The crowns are wider mesiodistally when compared with crown length than their permanent successors.

The roots are long and evenly tapered.

Although the dimensions are quite different, the functional design of the deciduous mandibular canine is similar to that of the maxillary canine. One variation which should be noted: the mandibular canine has its longest cusp slope to the distal, and the maxillary canine has its longest cusp slope to the mesial side. This makes for proper intercuspation of these teeth during mastication (Fig. 149).

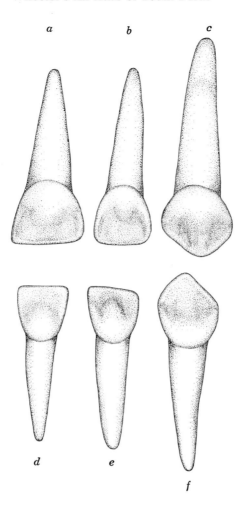

a   *b*   *c*

Figure 149. Deciduous right anterior teeth, lingual aspect. *a*, Maxillary central incisor; *b*, maxillary lateral incisor; *c*, maxillary canine; *d*, mandibular central incisor; *e*, mandibular lateral incisor; *f*, mandibular canine.

d   *e*

f

Lingual Aspects—Maxillary (Fig. 149 a, b, c)

The lingual aspects of the deciduous maxillary incisors show well-developed marginal ridges and highly developed cinguli. The cinguli extend up toward incisal ridges on lingual surfaces far enough to make partial divisions into mesial and distal fossae.

The roots are narrowed on the lingual surfaces, presenting relatively sharp ridges rootwise when compared to the broader, flattened labial surfaces.

The lingual aspect of the deciduous maxillary canine shows pronounced enamel ridges which merge with each other. They are the cingulum, mesial and distal marginal ridges and enamel ridges lingual to the cusp slopes. These ridges divide the lingual surface into two depressions or fossae.

The root of this tooth also tapers lingually.

Lingual Aspects—Mandibular (Fig. 149 d, e, f)

The lingual surfaces of the deciduous mandibular incisors have well-formed marginal ridges and cinguli. Some of these teeth will be quite flat and level between marginal ridges but some will show a decided concavity. The crowns taper lingually along with the roots so that the measurements lingually at the cervical third are narrower than those taken labially.

The lingual aspect of the deciduous mandibular canine varies from the mandibular incisors in these details: there is a cusp ridge from cingulum to cusp tip which may be pronounced enough to divide the lingual surface into defined fossae. The larger dimensions of the tooth give it a larger cingulum formation and a heavier, longer root.

Mesial and Distal Aspects—Maxillary (Fig. 150 a, b, c)

The mesial and distal aspects of deciduous maxillary incisors are similar. The measurement of both crowns at the cervical third shows them to be wide in relation to total crown length. This measurement on central incisors shows them to be only about 1 mm. less than the entire crown length cervicoincisally. From the mesial aspect deciduous anterior tooth crowns appear much thicker and more blunt than their permanent successors. The curvature of the cementoenamel junction on these crowns mesially and distally, although distinct, is much less than on permanent anterior teeth. The cervical ridges, which appear as distinct bulges of enamel at the cervical third, are much more prominent on all deciduous tooth crowns than on any of the crowns of permanent teeth. This is an important observation to be considered in operative procedures on deciduous teeth.

From the mesial aspect the outline form of the deciduous maxillary canine is similar to that of the central and lateral incisors, although there is considerable difference in proportions. The labiolingual measurement of the crown is usually greater than that of the crown length. This design, along with strong root anchorage, makes the tooth very serviceable when used in conjunction with the deciduous molars; besides assisting greatly in mastication, it offers good jaw support at all times.

Figure 150. Deciduous right anterior teeth, mesial aspect. *a*, Maxillary central incisor; *b*, maxillary lateral incisor; *c*, maxillary canine; *d*, mandibular central incisor; *e*, mandibular lateral incisor; *f*, mandibular canine.

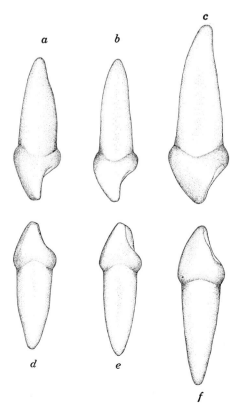

The roots of the deciduous maxillary incisors and canines appear more blunt from the mesial or distal aspects but, in general, they have a gradual taper toward the apical ends.

Mesial and Distal Aspects—Mandibular (Fig. 150 d, e, f)

The mesial and distal aspects of both the deciduous mandibular central incisor and the mandibular lateral incisor are similar. The mesial and distal aspects show the typical outline of incisor teeth even though the measurements are small. The incisal edges are centered over the roots and between the crown curvature labially and lingually. The convexity of the cervical contours labially and lingually at the cervical third is just as pronounced as in any of the other deciduous incisors and more so than the curvatures found at the same locations in permanent mandibular incisors. The crowns appear rather short cervicoincisally when compared with labiolingual width.

The roots appear long and evenly tapered from mesial and distal aspects.

When viewed from the mesial or distal aspect the deciduous mandibular canine exhibits little difference in functional form between this tooth and the deciduous maxillary canine. However, there is an outstanding variation in dimension. The tooth is much narrower labiolingually, making the tooth look much smaller than the maxillary canine from these aspects.

The root is evenly tapered from cementoenamel junction to apex.

Incisal (Occlusal) Aspects—Maxillary (Fig. 151 a, b, c)

An important feature to note when viewing deciduous maxillary incisors from the incisal aspect is the measurement mesiodistally with the measurement labiolingually. These measurements vary little. This makes the proportions different from permanent teeth, in which larger mesiodistal measurements make these teeth look more slender labiolingually.

The incisal edges are centered over the main bulk of the crowns and the edges are relatively straight. Looking down on the incisal edge, one sees that the labial surface is broader and smoother than that of the lingual surface. The lingual surface tapers toward the cingulum.

The deciduous maxillary canine appears very heavy and large when compared with other anterior teeth from the incisal aspect. It is distinctly diamond-shaped with evenly distributed bulk. The tapered sides of the crown appear to be even in every direction, mesially, distally, labially and lingually.

Incisal (Occlusal) Aspects—Mandibular (Fig. 151 d, e, f)

The incisal ridges of deciduous mandibular incisors are straight when viewed from the incisal aspect, and the ridges are placed so that they bisect the crowns labiolingually. The labial surfaces appear rather flat, perhaps a little to the convex, whereas the lingual surfaces show flattened areas slightly concave. The labial surfaces are relatively broad, the lingual surfaces tapering toward the cingulum.

A comparison of the incisal aspect of the deciduous mandibular canine with that of the maxillary canine shows the following: The deciduous mandibular canine is rounder on all surfaces and the crown is smaller. The lingual surface is smoother, with a tendency toward one lingual fossa,

Figure 151. Deciduous right anterior teeth, incisal aspect. *a*, Maxillary central incisor; *b*, maxillary lateral incisor; *c*, maxillary canine; *d*, mandibular central incisor; *e*, mandibular lateral incisor; *f*, mandibular canine.

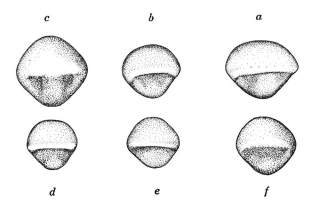

whereas the deciduous maxillary canine has a more uneven lingual surface with two lingual depressions divided by a heavy lingual ridge.

Molars

Buccal Aspect—Maxillary First Molar (Fig. 152 a)

The widest measurement of the crown of the deciduous maxillary first molar is at the contact areas mesially and distally. From these points the crown converges toward the cervix, the measurement at the cervix being fully 2 mm. less than the measurement at the contact areas. The occlusal line is slightly scalloped but with no definite cusp form. The buccal surface is smooth, and there is little evidence of developmental grooves.

The *roots* are slender and long, and they have a wide spread. All three roots may be seen from this aspect. The distal root is considerably shorter than the mesial. The *bifurcation* of the roots begins immediately above the cervical line of the crown. The bifurcation buccally on permanent molars is located some distance apical to the cervical line, so the permanent molars have a *root trunk* which shows greater development.

Buccal Aspect—Maxillary Second Molar (Fig. 152 b)

The deciduous maxillary second molar resembles the *permanent* maxillary first molar except in size. (Compare measurement tables.) Therefore, the buccal view of this tooth shows two well-defined buccal cusps with a buccal developmental groove between them. Characteristically, the crown is narrow at the cervix in comparison with its mesiodistal measurement at the contact areas. This crown is considerably larger than that of the first deciduous molar. Although the roots, from this aspect, appear slender, they are much longer and heavier than those found on the deciduous maxillary first molar. The point of bifurcation between the buccal roots is close to the cervical line of the crown. The two buccal cusps are more nearly equal in size and development than those of the deciduous maxillary first molar.

Buccal Aspect—Mandibular First Molar (Fig. 152 c)

This tooth does not resemble any of the other teeth, deciduous or permanent. Because it varies so much from all others, it appears strange and primitive (Figs. 154 *c*, and 156 *a*).

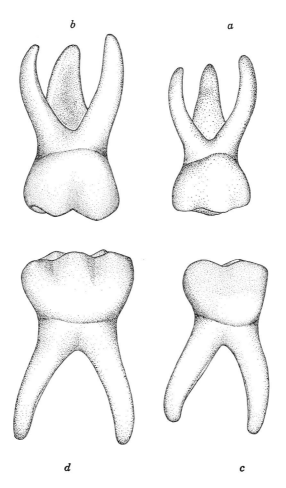

Figure 152. Deciduous right molars, buccal aspect. *a,* Maxillary first molar; *b,* maxillary second molar; *c,* mandibular first molar; *d,* mandibular second molar.

From the buccal aspect the mesial outline of the crown of the deciduous mandibular first molar is almost straight from the contact area to the cervix, constricting the crown very little at the cervix. The outline describing the distal portion, however, converges toward the cervix more than usual, making the contact area extend distally to a marked degree.

The distal portion of the crown is shorter than the mesial portion, the cervical line dipping apically where it joins the mesial root.

The two buccal cusps are rather distinct, although there is no developmental groove between them. The mesial cusp is larger than the distal cusp. There is a developmental depression dividing them, which extends over the buccal surface.

The roots are long and slender, and they spread greatly at the apical third beyond the outline of the crown.

As is characteristic of all deciduous molars, the point of bifurcation between the roots is very close to the cervical line of the crown.

Buccal Aspect—Mandibular Second Molar (Fig. 152 d)

The deciduous mandibular second molar resembles the permanent mandibular first molar except in its dimensions.

From the buccal aspect, the deciduous mandibular second molar has a mesiodistal measurement at the cervix much less in proportion to its mesiodistal measurement at the contact areas than that measurement on mandibular first permanent molars. A mesiobuccal and a distobuccal developmental groove divide the buccal surface occlusally into three cusps which are almost equal in size. This arrangement differs from the mandibular first permanent molar.

The roots of the deciduous second molar from this angle are slender and long. They have a characteristic flair mesiodistally at the middle and apical thirds. The roots of this tooth are usually twice as long as the crown, if not longer in proportion.

The point of bifurcation of the roots starts immediately below the cervical line of the crown buccally.

Lingual Aspect—Maxillary First Molar (Fig. 153 a)

The general outline of the lingual aspect of the crown is similar to the buccal aspect, although the crown converges considerably in a lingual direction.

The mesiolingual cusp is the most prominent cusp on this tooth. It is the longest and sharpest cusp. The distolingual cusp is poorly defined: it is small and rounded. From the lingual aspect the distobuccal cusp may be seen, since it is longer and better developed than the distolingual cusp. There is a type of deciduous maxillary first molar which is not uncommon and which presents one large lingual cusp with no developmental markings in evidence lingually. This type is apparently a three-cusped molar.

All three roots may be seen from this aspect also. The lingual root is larger than the others. Note the flair of roots extending their outlines beyond the measurement of crown outlines.

Lingual Aspect—Maxillary Second Molar (Fig. 153 b)

Lingually, the crown shows three cusps: (1) the mesiolingual cusp, which is large and well developed; (2), the distolingual cusp, which is also well developed (more so than that of the deciduous first molar), and (3) a third supplemental cusp, which is apical to the mesiolingual cusp and which is sometimes called the *tubercule of Carabelli* or the fifth cusp. This cusp is poorly developed and merely acts as a buttress or supplement to the bulk of the mesiolingual cusp. A well-defined developmental groove separates the mesiolingual cusp from the distolingual cusp and connects with the developmental groove which outlines the fifth cusp.

All three roots are visible from this aspect; the lingual root is large and thick in comparison with the other two roots. It is approximately the same length as the mesiobuccal root.

Lingual Aspect—Mandibular First Molar (Fig. 153 c)

The crown and root converge lingually to a marked degree on the mesial surface and this surface appears quite flat and straight. Distally, the opposite arrangement is true of both crown and root; the crown is, therefore, rhomboidal in outline. (See Fig. 156 a.) The mesiolingual cusp is long and sharp at the tip, sharper than any of the other cusps. It will be noted that the mesial marginal ridge is so well developed that it might almost be

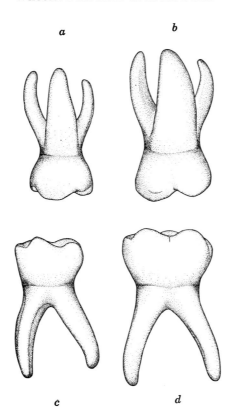

a   *b*

c   *d*

Figure 153. Deciduous right molars, lingual aspect. *a,* Maxillary first molar; *b,* maxillary second molar; *c,* mandibular first molar; *d,* mandibular second molar.

considered another small cusp as it approaches the lingual portion. Part of the two buccal cusps may be seen from this angle. The mesial root is thinner on the lingual side, the root being relatively straight and directly below the crown. The distal root is heavier and extends distally beyond the distal outline of the crown.

Lingual Aspect—Mandibular Second Molar (Fig. 153 d)

From the lingual aspect one sees two cusps of almost equal dimensions. Between them is a short lingual groove. The two lingual cusps are not quite so wide as the three buccal cusps; this arrangement narrows the crown lingually. The cervical line is relatively straight, and the crown extends out over the root about the same mesially as it does distally. A portion of each of the three buccal cusps may be seen from this aspect.

The roots from this aspect give somewhat the same appearance as from the buccal aspect. Note the length and flair of the roots.

Mesial Aspect—Maxillary First Molar (Fig. 154 a)

From the mesial aspect the measurement at the cervical third is greater than the measurement at the occlusal third. This is true of all molar forms, but it is more pronounced on deciduous teeth than on permanent teeth. The mesiolingual cusp is longer and sharper than the mesiobuccal cusp. There is a pronounced convexity in the buccal outline at the cervical third. This convexity is an outstanding characteristic of this tooth. Actually, it gives the impression of overdevelopment in this area when comparisons are made with any other tooth, deciduous or permanent. The remainder of the crown outline buccally is quite straight and flat as it approaches the occlusal surface. The lingual cusp form is sharper than the buccal cusp form.

The mesiobuccal and lingual roots are visible when one looks at the mesial side of this tooth from a point directly opposite the contact area. The distobuccal root is hidden behind the mesiobuccal root. The lingual root from this aspect looks long and slender and extends lingually to a marked degree. It curves sharply in a buccal direction above the middle third.

Mesial Aspect—Maxillary Second Molar (Fig. 154 b)

From the mesial aspect the crown has a typical molar outline and resembles that of the permanent molars. The crown appears short because of its width buccolingually in comparison with its length cervico-occlusally. The crown of this tooth is usually only about 0.5 mm. longer cervico-occlusally than the crown of the first deciduous molar, but the buccolingual measurement is 1.5 to 2 mm. greater. In addition, the roots are 1.5 to 2 mm. longer. The mesiolingual cusp of the crown with its supplementary fifth cusp appears large in comparison with the mesiobuccal cusp. The mesiobuccal cusp from this angle is relatively short and sharp. There is very

Figure 154. Deciduous right molars, mesial aspect. a, Maxillary first molar; b, maxillary second molar; c, mandibular first molar; d, mandibular second molar.

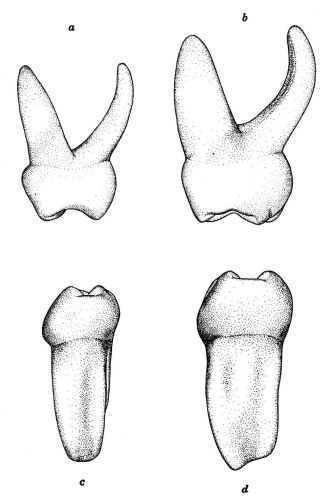

little curvature to the cervical line at the cementoenamel junction. Usually it is almost straight across from buccal surface to lingual surface.

The mesiobuccal root from this aspect appears broad and flat. The lingual root has somewhat the same curvature as the lingual root of the maxillary first deciduous molar. It extends lingually far out beyond the crown outline. The point of bifurcation between the mesiobuccal root and the lingual root is 2 or 3 mm. apical to the cervical line of the crown and approximately two-thirds the distance from buccal surface to lingual surface. The mesiolingual cusp is directly below this point. Although the curvature lingually on the crown from this aspect is great at the cervical portion, as on most deciduous teeth, the crest of curvature buccally at the cervical third is slight and resembles the curvature found at this point on the permanent maxillary first molar. In this it differs entirely from the accented curvature found on the deciduous maxillary first molars at the cervical third buccally. This is an important observation in operative procedure.

Mesial Aspect—Mandibular First Molar (Fig. 154 c)

The most noticeable detail from the mesial aspect is the extreme curvature buccally at the cervical third. Except for this detail, the crown outline of this tooth from this aspect is similar to the mesial aspect of the deciduous second molar and the permanent mandibular molars; the buccal cusps are placed over the root base, and the lingual outline of the crown extends out lingually beyond the confines of the root base.

Both the mesiobuccal cusp and the mesiolingual cusp are in view from this aspect, as is the well-developed mesial marginal ridge. Since the mesiobuccal crown length is greater than the mesiolingual crown length, the cervical line slants upward buccolingually. Note the flat appearance of the buccal outline of the crown from the crest of curvature of the buccal surface at the cervical third to the tip of the mesiobuccal cusp. All the deciduous molars have flattened buccal surfaces above this crest.

The outline of the mesial root from the mesial aspect does not resemble the outline of any other deciduous tooth root. The buccal and lingual outlines of the root drop straight down from the crown and are approximately parallel for over half their length, tapering only slightly at the apical third. The root end is flat and almost square. A developmental depression usually extends almost the full length of the root.

Mesial Aspect—Mandibular Second Molar (Fig. 154 d)

From the mesial aspect the outline of the crown resembles the permanent mandibular *first* molar. The variations are: the crest of contour buccally is more prominent on the deciduous molar; the tooth seems to be more constricted occlusally because of the flattened buccal surface above the crest of contour.

The crown has the characteristic position over the root of all mandibular posteriors, with its buccal cusp over the root and the lingual outline of the crown extending out beyond the root outline. The marginal ridge is high, a characteristic which makes the mesiobuccal cusp and the mesiolingual cusp appear rather short. The lingual cusp is longer, or extends higher at any rate, than the buccal cusp. The cervical line is regular, although it extends upward buccolingually, thereby making up for the difference in length between the buccal cusp and the lingual cusp.

The mesial root is very broad and flat.

Distal Aspect—Maxillary First Molar

From the distal aspect the crown is narrower distally than mesially. The distobuccal cusp is long and sharp, and the distolingual cusp is poorly developed. The prominence seen from the mesial aspect at the cervical third does not continue distally. The cervical line may curve occlusally, or it may extend straight across from the buccal surface to the lingual surface. All three roots may be seen from this angle, but the distobuccal root is superimposed on the mesiobuccal root so that only the buccal surface and the apex of the latter may be seen. The point of bifurcation of the distobuccal root and the lingual root is more apical to the cervical line at this point than the points of bifurcation described heretofore.

Distal Aspect—Maxillary Second Molar

From the distal aspect it is apparent that the distal measurement of the crown is less than the mesial measurement, but not to the degree found on the deciduous maxillary first molar. From both the distal and the mesial aspects the outline of the crown lingually appears almost semicircular, whereas a line describing the buccal surface is almost straight from the crest of curvature to the occlusal surface. The distobuccal cusp and the distolingual cusp are about the same in length. The cervical line is approximately straight, as was found mesially.

All three roots are seen from this aspect, although only a part of the outline of the mesiobuccal root may be seen, since the distobuccal root is superimposed over it. The distobuccal root is shorter and narrower than the other roots. The point of bifurcation between the distobuccal root and the lingual root is more apical in position that any of the other points of bifurcation. The point of bifurcation between these two roots on the distal is more nearly centered above the crown than that on the mesial between the mesiobuccal and lingual roots.

Distal Aspect—Mandibular First Molar

The distal aspect of the mandibular first molar differs from the mesial aspect as follows: There is less curvature at the cervical third buccally. The length of crown buccally and lingually is more uniform, and the cervical line extends almost straight across buccolingually. The distobuccal cusp and the distolingual cusp are not so long nor so sharp as the two mesial cusps. The distal marginal ridge is not so well defined as the mesial marginal ridge. The distal root is rounder and shorter and tapers more apically.

Distal Aspect—Mandibular Second Molar

The crown is not so wide distally as it is mesially; therefore, it is possible to see the mesiobuccal cusp as well as the distobuccal cusp from the distal aspect. The distolingual cusp appears well developed, and the triangular ridge from the tip of this cusp extending down into the occlusal surface is seen over the distal marginal ridge.

The distal marginal ridge dips down more sharply and is shorter buccolingually than the mesial marginal ridge. The cervical line of the crown is regular, although it has the same upward incline buccolingually on the distal as on the mesial.

The distal root is almost as broad as the mesial root, and it is flattened on the distal surface. The distal root tapers more at the apical end than does the mesial root.

Occlusal Aspect—Maxillary First Molar (Fig. 155 a)

The calibration of the distance between the mesiobuccal line angle and the distobuccal line angle is definitely greater than that found between the mesiolingual line angle and the distolingual line angle. This makes the crown outline converge lingually. Also, the calibration from the mesiobuccal line angle to the mesiolingual line angle is definitely greater than that found at both distal line angles. Therefore, the crown converges distally also. Nevertheless, the occlusal surface as outlined by the cusp tips and marginal ridges does not show this convergence. The occlusal surface is more nearly rectangular, with the shortest sides of the rectangle represented by the marginal ridges.

The occlusal surface has a *central fossa*. There is a *mesial triangular fossa*, just inside the mesial marginal ridge, with a mesial pit in this fossa and a sulcus with its *central groove* connecting the two fossae. There is also a well-defined *buccal developmental groove* dividing the mesiobuccal cusp and the distobuccal cusp occlusally. There are supplemental grooves radiating from the pit in the mesial triangular fossa. These grooves radiate as follows: one buccally, one lingually and one toward the marginal ridge, the last sometimes extending over the marginal ridge mesially.

Sometimes the deciduous maxillary first molar has a well-defined triangular ridge connecting the mesiolingual cusp with the distobuccal cusp. When well developed, it is called the *oblique ridge*. In some of these teeth the ridge will be very indefinite and the central developmental groove will extend from the mesial pit to the *disto-occlusal groove*. This disto-occlusal groove is always seen and may or may not extend through to the lingual surface, outlining a distolingual cusp. The distal marginal ridge is thin and poorly developed in comparison with the mesial marginal ridge.

Summary of the Occlusal Aspect of This Tooth

The form of the maxillary first deciduous molar varies from that of any tooth in the permanent dentition. Although there are no premolars in the deciduous set, in some respects the crown of this deciduous molar resembles a permanent maxillary premolar. Nevertheless, the divisions of the occlusal surface and the root form with its efficient anchorage make it a molar, both in type and function.

Occlusal Aspect—Maxillary Second Molar (Fig. 155 b)

From the occlusal aspect this tooth resembles the permanent first molar. It is somewhat rhomboidal and has four well-developed cusps and one supplemental cusp: mesiobuccal, distobuccal, mesiolingual, distolingual and fifth cusp. The buccal surface is rather flat, with the developmental groove between the cusps less marked than that found on the first permanent molar. Developmental grooves, pits, oblique ridge, etc., are almost identical.

The occlusal surface has a *central fossa* with a *central pit*, a well-defined *mesial triangular fossa*, just distal to the *mesial marginal ridge*, with a

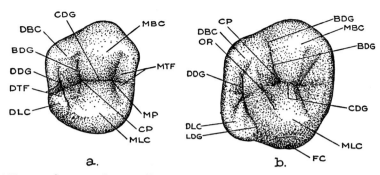

Figure 155. Deciduous right maxillary molars, occlusal aspect. *a*, First molar. *MBC*, Mesiobuccal cusp; *MTF*, mesial triangular fossa; *MP*, mesial pit; *CP*, central pit; *MLC*, mesiolingual cusp; *DLC*, distolingual cusp; *DTF*, distal triangular fossa; *DDG*, distal developmental groove; *BDG*, buccal developmental groove; *DBC*, distobuccal cusp; *CDG*, central developmental groove.

b, Second molar. *BDG*, Buccal developmental groove; *MBC*, mesiobuccal cusp; *CDG*, central developmental groove; *MLC*, mesiolingual cusp; *FC*, fifth cusp; *LDG*, lingual developmental groove; *DLC*, distolingual cusp; *DDG*, distal developmental groove; *OR*, oblique ridge; *DBC*, distobuccal cusp; *CP*, central pit.

mesial pit at its center. There is, too, a well-defined developmental groove called the *central groove* at the bottom of a sulcus connecting the mesial triangular fossa with the central fossa. The *buccal developmental groove* extends buccally from the central pit, separating the triangular ridges which are occlusal continuations of the mesio- and distobuccal cusps. Supplemental grooves often radiate from these developmental grooves.

The *oblique ridge* is prominent and connects the mesiolingual cusp with the distobuccal cusp. Distal to the oblique ridge one finds the *distal fossa*, which harbors the *distal developmental groove*. The distal groove has branches of supplemental grooves within the *distal triangular fossa*, which is rather indefinitely outlined just mesial to the distal marginal ridge.

The distal groove acts as a line of demarcation between the mesiolingual and distolingual cusps and continues on to the lingual surface as the *lingual developmental groove*. The *distal marginal ridge* is as well developed as the *mesial marginal ridge*. It will be remembered that the marginal ridges are not developed equally on the deciduous maxillary first molar.

Occlusal Aspect—Mandibular First Molar (Fig. 156 a)

The deciduous mandibular first molar does not resemble any of the other teeth, deciduous or permanent; this is particularly noticeable from the occlusal aspect. Because it varies so much from the others, it appears strange and primitive. The general outline of this tooth from the occlusal aspect is rhomboidal. The prominence mesiobuccally at the cervical third is noticeable from this aspect also, a fact which accents the mesiobuccal line angle of the crown in comparison with the distobuccal line angle.

The mesiolingual cusp may be seen as the largest and the best developed of all the cusps, and it has a broad flattened surface lingually. The *buccal developmental groove* of the occlusal surface divides the two buccal cusps evenly. This developmental groove is short, extending from between the buccal cusp ridges to a point approximately in the center of the crown outline at a *central pit*. The *central developmental groove* joins it at this point and extends mesially, separating the mesiobuccal cusp and the mesiolingual cusp. The central groove ends in a *mesial pit* in the *mesial triangular fossa* which is immediately distal to the *mesial marginal ridge*. Two supplemental grooves join the developmental groove in the center of the mesial triangular fossa; one supplemental groove extends buccally and the other extends lingually.

The mesiobuccal cusp exhibits a well-defined triangular ridge on the occlusal surface which terminates in the center of the occlusal surface buccolingually at the *central developmental groove*. Another triangular ridge extends lingually from this point, joining with the mesiolingual cusp. Usually a lingual developmental groove does not extend through to the lingual surface but stops at the junction of lingual cusp ridges. There are some supplemental grooves immediately mesial to the *distal marginal ridge* in the *distal triangular fossa* which join with the central developmental groove.

Occlusal Aspect—Mandibular Second Molar (Fig. 156 b)

The occlusal aspect of the deciduous mandibular second molar is somewhat rectangular. The three buccal cusps are similar in size. Thus, it differs from the *permanent* mandibular *first* molar, which it resembles in other ways. The two lingual cusps are equally matched. However, the total mesiodistal width of the lingual cusps is less than the total mesiodistal width of the three buccal cusps.

There are well-defined triangular ridges extending occlusally from each one of these cusp tips. The triangular ridges end in the center of the crown buccolingually in a *central developmental groove* which follows a staggered course from the *mesial triangular fossa*, just inside the *mesial marginal ridge*, to the *distal triangular fossa*, just mesial to the *distal marginal ridge*. The distal triangular fossa is not so well defined as the mesial triangular fossa. Developmental grooves branch off from the central groove both buccally and lingually, dividing the cusps. The two *buccal grooves* are

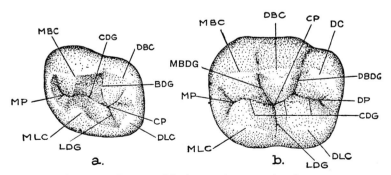

Figure 156. Deciduous right mandibular molars, occlusal aspect *a*, First molar. *CDG*, Central developmental groove; *DBC*, distobuccal cusp; *BDG*, buccal developmental groove; *CP*, central pit; *DLC*, distolingual cusp; *LDG*, lingual developmental groove; *MLC*, mesiolingual cusp; *MP*, mesial pit; *MBC*, mesiobuccal cusp.

b, Second molar. *DBC*, Distobuccal cusp; *CP*, central pit; *DC*, distal cusp; *DBDG*, distobuccal developmental groove; *DP*, distal pit; *CDG*, central developmental groove; *DLC*, distolingual cusp; *LDG*, lingual developmental groove; *MLC*, mesiolingual cusp; *MP*, mesial pit; *MBDG*, mesiobuccal developmental groove; *MBC*, mesiobuccal cusp.

confluent with the buccal developmental grooves of the buccal surface, one *mesial* and one *distal*, and the single *lingual developmental groove* is confluent with the *lingual groove* on the lingual surface of the crown.

Scattered over the occlusal surface are supplemental grooves on the slopes of triangular ridges and in the mesial and distal triangular fossae. The mesial marginal ridge is better developed and more pronounced than the distal marginal ridge. The outline of the crown converges distally. An outline following the tips of the cusps and the marginal ridges conforms to the outline of a rectangle more closely than does the gross outline of the crown in its entirety.

A comparison between the *deciduous mandibular second molar* and the *permanent mandibular first molar* brings out the following points of difference: The deciduous molar has its mesiobuccal, distobuccal and distal cusps almost equal in size and development. The distal cusp of the permanent molar is smaller than the other two. Because of the small buccal cusps, the deciduous tooth crown is narrower buccolingually, in comparison with its mesiodistal measurement, than is the permanent tooth.

THE OCCLUSION OF THE DECIDUOUS TEETH

The deciduous teeth are arranged in the jaws in the form of two arches: a maxillary arch and a mandibular arch (Fig. 157). An outline following the labial and buccal surfaces of the maxillary teeth describes the segment of an ellipse, an outline which is larger than the segment following the same surfaces on the mandibular teeth.

The relation between the maxillary and mandibular deciduous teeth when in occlusion is such that each tooth, with the exception of the mandibular central incisor and the maxillary second molar, occludes with two teeth of the opposite jaw. The deciduous teeth should be in normal alignment, contact and occlusion shortly after the age of two, with all the roots fully formed by the time the child is three years old. A year or so after the teeth have fully erupted and have assumed their respective positions in the arches, the rapid development of the jaws is sufficient to create a slight space, or diastema, between some of them.

In this manner, the anterior teeth separate and usually show more separation as time goes on—a process which is caused by the approach of the permanent teeth from the lingual side in addition to jaw growth. The canines and molars are supposed to keep their positive contact relation during all the jaw growth. However, some shifting and separation of these teeth may take place. When the teeth do not hold their relative positions, they are worn off rapidly on incisal ridges and occlusal surfaces. As an example, when a deciduous canine is lost eight years or more after its eruption, its long, sharp cusp has usually been worn flat. If the deciduous teeth are in good alignment, the occlusion is most efficient during the time that these teeth are in their original positions.

After normal jaw growth has caused considerable separation, the occlusion is supported and made more efficient by the eruption and occlusion of the first permanent molars immediately distal to the deciduous second molars. The child is now approximately six years of age, and he will use some of his deciduous teeth for six more years. This period is sometimes called the mixed dentition period (Fig. 158).

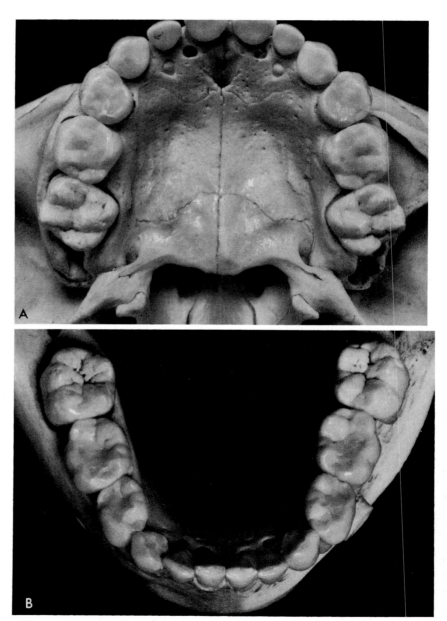

Figure 157. Deciduous dentition with first permanent molars present.

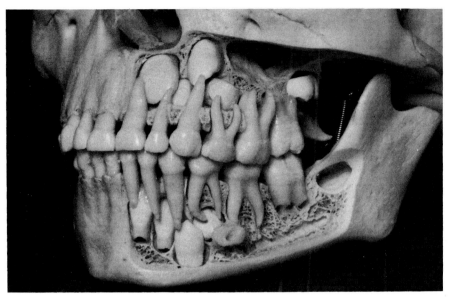

Figure 158. Mixed dentition with first permanent molars in position (artifactual loss of mandibular molar from crypt).

Details of Occlusion (Fig. 159)

The occlusion of deciduous teeth, in a three-year-old child, may be described. After separation has begun, the migration of the teeth changes the occlusion. Nevertheless, if development is normal, the spacing of the teeth is rather uniform.

Normal occlusion of deciduous teeth at the age of three years is as follows:

1. Mesial surfaces of maxillary and mandibular central incisors are in line with each other at the median line.

2. The maxillary central incisor occludes with the mandibular central incisor and the mesial third of the mandibular lateral incisor. The mandibular

Figure 159. Occlusal surface of the mandibular deciduous teeth in child three years of age, with the outlines of the opposing teeth superposed in occlusion (Freil, Internat. J. Orthodontia and Oral Surgery).

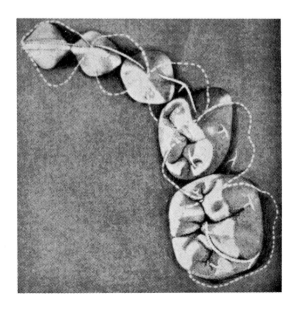

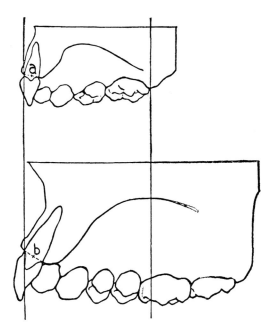

Figure 160. Drawing of a sagittal section through the permanent and deciduous maxillary incisors. The labial surface at the cervical margin is oriented in the same plane. Note that the midalveolar point of the permanent incisors, *b*, is more lingual than the midalveolar point of the deciduous incisors, *a*, but that the incisal edge of the permanent incisors is more labial than that of the deciduous incisors (Freil, Internat. J. Orthodontia and Oral Surgery).

anterior teeth strike the maxillary anterior teeth lingually above the level of the incisal ridges.

3. The maxillary lateral incisor occludes with the distal two-thirds of the mandibular lateral incisor and that portion of the mandibular canine which is mesial to the point of its cusp.

4. The maxillary canine occludes with that portion of the mandibular canine distal to its cusp tip and the mesial third of the mandibular first molar (that portion mesial to the tip of the mesiobuccal cusp).

5. The maxillary first molar occludes with the distal two-thirds of the mandibular first molar and the mesial portion of the mandibular second molar, which portion is represented by the mesial marginal ridge and the mesial triangular fossa.

6. The maxillary second molar occludes with the remainder of the mandibular second molar, the distal surface of the maxillary molar projecting slightly over the distal portion of the mandibular second molar.

The interrelation of cusps and incisal ridges of the opposing arches of deciduous teeth may be studied in the illustrations by Sheldon Freil. The relation in size of deciduous and permanent arches is also illustrated by him in Figure 160.